DERMOSCOPY
The Essentials

Commissioning Editor: Sue Hodgson
Project Development Manager: Tim Kimber
Project Manager: Camilla Rockwood/Glenys Norquay
Design Manager: Jayne Jones

DERMOSCOPY
The Essentials

Robert Johr MD
Clinical Professor of Dermatology and Pediatrics,
Director Pigmented Lesion Clinic,
University of Miami School of Medicine,
Miami, Florida, USA

H. Peter Soyer MD
Professor of Dermatology,
Department of Dermatology,
Medical University of Graz,
Graz, Austria

Giuseppe Argenziano MD
Assistant Professor of Dermatology,
Department of Dermatology,
Second University of Naples,
Naples, Italy

Rainer Hofmann-Wellenhof MD
Professor of Dermatology,
Department of Dermatology,
Medical University of Graz,
Graz, Austria

Massimiliano Scalvenzi MD
Assistant Professor of Dermatology,
Department of Dermatology,
University Federico II of Naples,
Naples, Italy

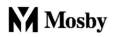 **Mosby**

Edinburgh London New York Oxford Philadelphia St Louis Sydney Toronto 2004

MOSBY

An imprint of Elsevier Limited

First published 2004
  Reprinted 2004, 2005 (twice), 2006, 2007

ISBN-13: 978–0–3230–2896–7
ISBN-10: 0–3230–2896–9

British Library Cataloguing in Publication Data
A catalogue record for this book is available from the British Library

Library of Congress Cataloging in Publication Data
A catalogue record for this book is available from the Library of Congress

Note
Medical knowledge is constantly changing. As new information becomes available, changes in treatment, procedures, equipment and the use of drugs become necessary. The author, contributor and the publishers have, as far as it is possible, taken care to ensure that the information given in this text is accurate and up to date. However, readers are strongly advised to confirm that the information, especially with regard to drug usage, complies with the latest legislation and standards of practice.

The Publisher

 ELSEVIER your source for books, journals and multimedia in the health sciences
www.elsevierhealth.com

Working together to grow libraries in developing countries
www.elsevier.com | www.bookaid.org | www.sabre.org
ELSEVIER   BOOK AID International   Sabre Foundation

The publisher's policy is to use **paper manufactured from sustainable forests**

Printed in China

Contents

Foreword

I wish to congratulate Drs Johr *et al* on their new and exciting text, *Dermoscopy – The Essentials*. I use dermoscopy every day in my dermatology practice, and continue to learn. I have read every page of this text, viewed every image, and I can only say that the learning curve was excellent for me! I believe that skin surface microscopy (dermoscopy) is the bridge between our standard clinical evaluation of pigmented lesions and the histopathological interpretation of those lesions when biopsied. Hence, dermoscopy is an extension of our standard visual diagnosis, wherein we can see through the lesion and not just the surface of the lesion. I believe that our international colleagues, especially those in Europe and Australia, are far ahead of most of us in the United States in terms of learning this technique and incorporating it into our clinical practice.

I hope that this well organized and superbly illustrated book will become a standard teaching text in dermatology programs throughout North America and the rest of the world. I believe that the teaching of skin surface microscopy is a neglected element in most programs in the USA.

I wanted to point out a little about the organization of the text and the reason why it teaches us so well. *Dermoscopy – The Essentials* breaks down the art of dermoscopy into bite-sized pieces that can be understood and remembered: the three-point check list, global pattern analysis, parallel patterns for melanocytic lesions, melanoma-specific local criteria, site-specific melanoma-specific criteria and criteria for diagnosing non-melanocytic lesions. Additional insight is also given into the diagnosis of pediatric lesions, interpreting black lesions, interpreting lesions in dark-skinned races, facial lesions (both nodular and flat), featureless melanomas (a real fright!), and mucosal lesions. Each of these packets of information is given in a concise manner, reinforced by multiple illustrations, so that the points are clearly driven home. The repetition is excellent reinforcement and not overdone. The quality of the images is outstanding. I learned something from virtually every page!

Why is dermoscopy the now neglected art that it is in North America? First of all, I think we have so few practitioners who truly understand it and incorporate it into their practice. Hence, dermatology residents are not exposed to it. If we count the numbers of hours spent in honing our standard visual diagnosis skills, and our acquisition of dermatopathological knowledge, these exercises would represent dozens of hours per week for each dermatology resident. Yet almost nowhere does a dermatology resident spend even one hour a week (perhaps other than in Miami with Dr Johr!) learning the features of dermoscopy. And yet, it is very learnable and teachable. I believe we are now developing a nucleus of people who can begin to teach this art. I have learned it both on my own, and also under the patient guidance of Dr Johr. We have invited him twice to Arizona to teach us this discipline; however, it must be taught over a much longer period of time and with much greater virtually daily reinforcement to really get the job done. I think this textbook can serve as a self-teaching module for practicing dermatologists and for dermatology programs. I think it will kick start many of us into using dermoscopy in our practices.

There are other reasons why dermoscopy has not prospered in this country. One is the honest concern that relying too strongly on dermoscopic criteria might prevent needed biopsy of a melanoma, putting the patient at risk, as well as the doctor. However, it is clear that skilled dermoscopists are much more discriminating with pigmented lesions, and are actually likely to see high risk features in cases where conventional examination would miss the high risk clues. The admonition 'when in doubt, cut it out' rings throughout this text. I personally see pediatric patients every day where dermoscopy relieves me and the family of concern about nevi and saves a child a biopsy. I am also frequently surprised by significant dermoscopic atypia with fairly bland clinical features.

In addition, there are economic and turf protection issues involved in the acceptance of dermoscopy. One will do fewer biopsies overall as an avid dermoscopist could spend more time evaluating the lesion. This means lost compensation since insurance does not reimburse for dermoscopy. Pathologists will receive fewer specimens. I am sure that these issues are important barriers to acceptance of skin surface microscopy. However, I am sure that we are more accurate in our decision making when we use dermoscopy, hence it is best for our patients. Dr Johr and his international colleagues have it right and their book will make it easier for the rest of us to learn this useful technique.

I have consistently used dermoscopy for the last four years in evaluating both adult and pediatric patients with pigmented problems. I now find it essential. I also have found the magnification useful to evaluate such important features as nail fold capillary telangectasia/dilated capillary loops in rheumatological disorders, hair shaft abnormalities,

observing scabies mites and closer inspection of congenital lesions such as nevus sebaceous. However, even in pediatric patients I mainly use dermoscopy to separate out concerning pigmented lesions from less concerning pigmented lesions. I follow two children with xeroderma pigmentosum, and have found it essential to separate out their numerous basal cell carcinomas from concerning melanocytic lesions. I have been able to make that separation in virtually all cases using dermoscopy patterns described in *Dermoscopy – The Essentials.*

My congratulations once again to the authors. I hope that the word spreads and dermoscopy becomes part of our visual diagnosis skill set. *Dermoscopy – The Essentials* should become an essential text for our profession.

Ronald C. Hansen MD
Chief of Pediatric Dermatology,
Phoenix Children's Hospital,
Phoenix, Arizona, USA

Preface

The authors of this book are on a quest. For years we have been lecturing, creating articles, CDs and books with the goal of making dermoscopy, dermatoscopy, epiluminescence microscopy, ELM, skin surface microscopy, or whatever you choose to call the technique, the standard of care for all dermatologists and others who see patients with pigmented skin lesions. There are wonderful works already written in the standard fashion that promote dermoscopy, yet in some way they have not lit a fire in us all to joyfully and relatively effortlessly learn a technique that spares tissue and saves lives.

If there are books that can teach languages such as German or Italian in '10 minutes a day' why not create a dermoscopy book that is 'short and sweet', '101', fun and easy to go through? The aim is to include images that cover everything that is out there, not only in a university clinic but also in private practice, and with facts that are the essentials and more!

This is not a classic medical textbook and that is intentional. For example, the 'traffic lights' are a tool for the busy practitioner to use to rapidly review the book over and over again, because one aspect of mastering dermoscopy is the internalization of the basic principles. Look at the images, then look at the colors of the traffic lights. Red indicates high-risk lesions, green for low-risk lesions and orange for the gray-zone lesions. The associations between what you see with dermoscopy and the traffic light colors will sink into the recesses of your mind and come into play when you see similar dermoscopic criteria or patterns on your patients. You have to learn the basics; however, intuition and 'gut' feelings come into play on a regular basis. Never ignore instinctive impressions.

We worked very well together as a team but it was not always easy, especially since the authors live on different continents and we face the typical trials and tribulations of the human experience. However, we never lost sight of our goal and egos did not take hold. This book is a work of love from doctors who are true believers in a technique that is essential for our patients. People's fathers, mothers, sons, daughters, grandparents, aunts, and uncles entrust us with their health, their lives! We have the responsibility to be the best that we can be to prevent the pain and suffering that goes along with the most insidious of enemies, melanoma. Let dermoscopy be like the seat belt of your car. You should never leave home without it.

The Authors

KEY TO TRAFFIC LIGHT SYMBOLS

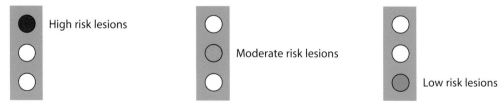

Acknowledgments

I have the best of both worlds – a very enjoyable private practice and the exciting world of academic dermatology at the University of Miami. This has been made possible by the person who runs my private office. Over the years she has allowed me to be free of mind to concentrate on being the best dermatologist I could be. She is my confidante, best friend and biggest supporter, my wife Irma. Without her instinctive common sense and help there are many other roads I would have taken in my life. I owe her a lot.

I would also like to thank my mentor and good friend, a master in the world of pediatric dermatology, Dr Lawrence Schachner. One of the greatest joys in my life is my association with the University of Miami. It has been a naturally evolving relationship and he has been instrumental in making that happen. I would not change that for the world.

Robert Johr

Special thanks go to my chairman Helmut Kerl, who has continuously supported my work on dermoscopy over the past two decades. He did it at a time when it was not apparent that dermoscopy would become such an important technique for the early diagnosis of melanoma.

H. Peter Soyer

I would like to acknowledge the great support given by Iris Zalaudek and Gianluca Petrillo for the accomplishment of this endeavor. In particular, Iris Zalaudek was responsible for the collection of part of the image database and Gianluca Petrillo did the digital imaging. A big thank you to them for their vital work! We are all in debt to Sue Hodgson and Tim Kimber for their great support. Particularly, they rendered things 'smoother' when many theoretical and practical problems related to the book were coming up. Finally, to my father, my first teacher and the best one. I learned from him the most important lessons: the curiosity, the love for a continuous search, the passion and dedication that are necessary to achieve your aims.

Giuseppe Argenziano

I would like to thank H. Peter Soyer for his excellent teaching in dermoscopy and the other co-authors, who made working on the book an exciting event in my scientific life. I would also like to thank Dr Iris Zalaudek for her great support and enthusiasm in taking wonderful dermoscopic images. Special thanks go to my wife and children, who have given me the strength to joyfully work on the book.

Rainer Hofmann-Wellenhof

Introduction – the 3-point checklist

The short, easy way to avoid missing a melanoma using dermoscopy

Dermoscopy is an in-vivo noninvasive diagnostic technique that magnifies the skin in such a way that color and structure in the epidermis, dermo-epidermal junction and papillary dermis become visible. This color and structure cannot be seen with the naked eye or with the typical magnification used by clinicians. With training and experience dermoscopy has been shown to significantly increase the clinical diagnosis of melanocytic, nonmelanocytic, benign and malignant skin lesions, with a 10–27% improvement in the diagnosis of melanoma compared to that achieved by clinical examination alone. There is, however, a learning curve to mastering dermoscopy and it is essential to spend time perfecting it – practice makes perfect!

OTHER NAMES FOR DERMOSCOPY
Dermatoscopy
Epiluminescence microscopy (ELM)
Skin surface microscopy
Auflichtmikroskopie
Digital dermoscopy, or digital ELM (DELM)

TECHNIQUE

In classic dermoscopy, oil or fluid (mineral oil, immersion oil, KY jelly, alcohol, water) is placed over the lesion to be examined. Fluid eliminates surface light reflection and renders the stratum corneum transparent, allowing visualization of subsurface colors and structures.

The list of dermoscopy instrumentation is long and continues to grow and evolve with the development of better and more sophisticated handheld instruments and computer systems. Depending on the budget and goals for the evaluation and management of patients with pigmented skin lesions, there is a wide variety of products to choose from.

THE 3-POINT CHECKLIST

To encourage clinicians to start using dermoscopy, simplified algorithms for analyzing what is seen with the technique have been developed.

For the novice dermoscopist, the primary goal of dermoscopy is to determine whether a suspicious lesion should be biopsied or excised. The bottom line is that no patient should leave the clinic with an undiagnosed melanoma.

For the general physician, dermoscopy can be used to determine whether a suspicious lesion should be evaluated by a more experienced clinician.

Dermoscopy is not just for dermatologists; any clinician who is interested can master this potentially life-saving technique.

TRIAGE OF SUSPICIOUS PIGMENTED SKIN LESIONS

The 3-point checklist was developed specifically for novice dermoscopists with little training to help them not to misdiagnose melanoma while improving their skills.

Results of the 2001 Consensus Net Meeting on Dermoscopy (Argenziano G, Soyer HP, Chimenti S et al. Dermoscopy of pigmented skin lesions: results of a consensus meeting via the internet. J Am Acad Dermatol 2003;48:679–93) showed that the following three criteria were especially important in distinguishing melanoma from other benign pigmented skin lesions:

- dermoscopic asymmetry of color and structure;
- atypical pigment network; and
- blue-white structures (a combination of the earlier categories of blue-white veil and regression structures).

Statistical analysis showed that the presence of any two of these criteria indicates a high likelihood of melanoma. Using the 3-point checklist one can have a sensitivity and specificity result comparable with other algorithms requiring much more training. In a preliminary study of 231 clinically equivocal pigmented skin lesions it was shown that after a short introduction of one-hour duration six inexperienced dermoscopists were able to classify 96.3% of melanomas correctly using this method.

This first chapter provides 60 examples of benign and malignant pigmented skin lesions to demonstrate how the 3-point checklist works and the practical value of this new and simplified diagnostic algorithm.

The 3-point checklist was designed to be used as a screening method. The sensitivity is much higher than the specificity to ensure that melanomas are not misdiagnosed. We recommend that all lesions with a positive test (3-point checklist score of 2 or 3) are excised.

3-POINT CHECKLIST	DEFINITION
1. Asymmetry	Asymmetry of color and structure in one or two perpendicular axes
2. Atypical network	Pigment network with irregular holes and thick lines
3. Blue-white structures	Any type of blue and/or white color

Table 1 Definition of dermoscopic criteria for the 3-point checklist. The presence of two or three criteria is suggestive of a suspicious lesion.

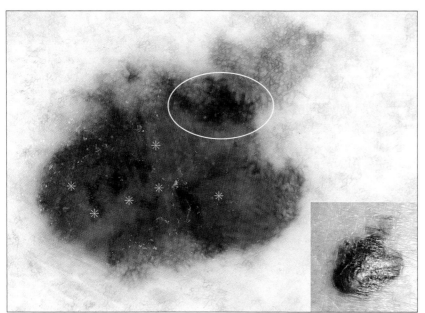
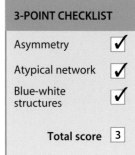

3-POINT CHECKLIST	
Asymmetry	✓
Atypical network	✓
Blue-white structures	✓
Total score	3

Figure 1   Melanoma

Criteria to diagnose melanoma can be very subtle or obviously present as in this case. This lesion clearly demonstrates all of the 3-point checklist criteria, namely, asymmetry in all axes, an atypical pigment network (circle) and blue-white structures (asterisks).

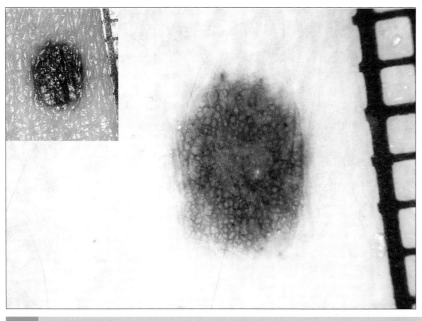

3-POINT CHECKLIST	
Asymmetry	☐
Atypical network	☐
Blue-white structures	☐
Total score	0

Figure 2   Nevus

In contrast to Figure 1, none of the features of the 3-point checklist are seen in this lesion. The lesion is symmetrical and the pigment network is regular although it might seem to be atypical because the line segments are slightly thickened.

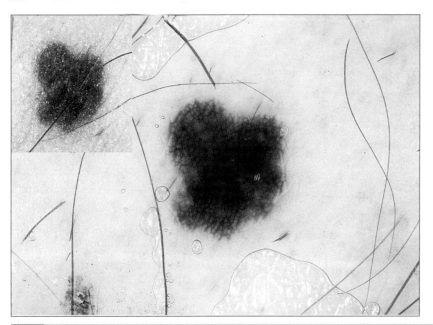

3-POINT CHECKLIST

Asymmetry	✔
Atypical network	☐
Blue-white structures	☐
Total score	1

Figure 3 Nevus

The novice might find this lesion difficult to diagnose. If in doubt cut it out! With experience the clinician will excise fewer of these banal nevi. There is asymmetry; however, it is questionable whether an atypical pigment network or subtle blue-white structures are present.

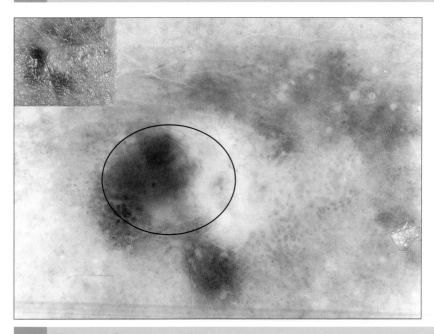
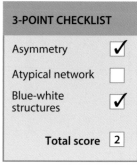

3-POINT CHECKLIST

Asymmetry	✔
Atypical network	☐
Blue-white structures	✔
Total score	2

Figure 4 Melanoma

Even for a beginner, the asymmetry of color and structure should be obvious. This strikingly asymmetrical lesion also demonstrates blue-white structures (circle).

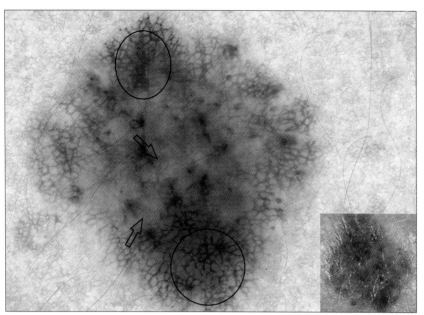

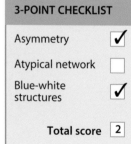

3-POINT CHECKLIST

Asymmetry	✔
Atypical network	✔
Blue-white structures	✔
Total score	3

Figure 5 Melanoma
The color and structure in the lower half is not a mirror image of the upper half; therefore there is asymmetry. An atypical pigment network with thickened and broken up line segments (circles) and a large area of blue-white structures (arrows) are also seen.

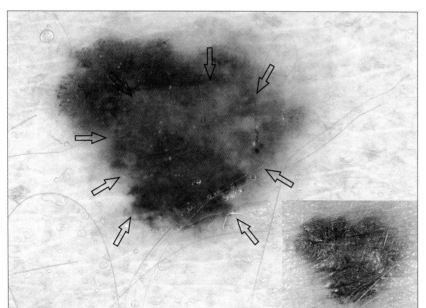

3-POINT CHECKLIST

Asymmetry	✔
Atypical network	
Blue-white structures	✔
Total score	2

Figure 6 Melanoma
A lesion like this one should immediately raise a red flag because there is a great deal of asymmetry of color and structure. No pigment network is present, but well developed blue-white structures (encircled by arrows) are seen in more than half of the lesion.

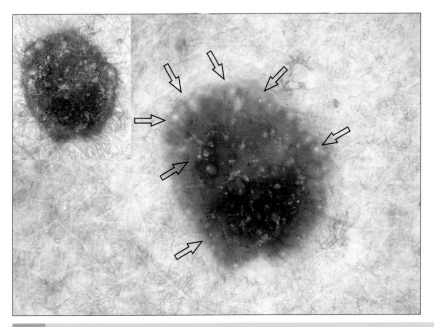

3-POINT CHECKLIST

Asymmetry	✔
Atypical network	☐
Blue-white structures	☐
Total score	1

Figure 7 Seborrheic keratosis
This seborrheic keratosis demonstrates a great deal of asymmetry of color and structure, but the other two criteria needed to diagnose melanoma are absent. If the multiple milia-like cysts (arrows) diagnostic of seborrheic keratosis cannot be recognized, excise the lesion.

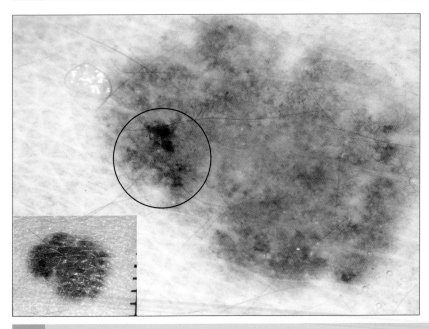

3-POINT CHECKLIST

Asymmetry	✔
Atypical network	☐
Blue-white structures	☐
Total score	1

Figure 8 Nevus
Some melanomas are featureless, so beware! The color and structure in the right half of the lesion is not a mirror image of the left half. The presence of irregular black dots in the left upper corner (circle) add to the asymmetry. Pigment network and blue-white structures are not seen.

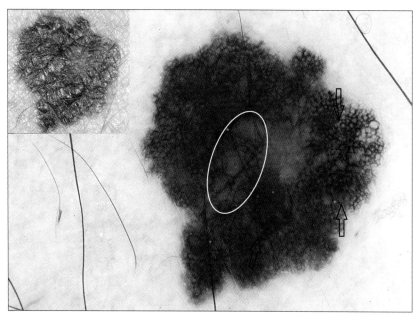

3-POINT CHECKLIST	
Asymmetry	☐
Atypical network	☐
Blue-white structures	☐
Total score	0

Figure 9   Nevus

If in doubt cut it out! With practice fewer lesions that look like this will be excised. This is highly symmetrical and there is a great example of a regular pigment network in this banal nevus. Do not be fooled by the dark central color – it is not always a sign of malignancy. No blue-white structures are seen.

3-POINT CHECKLIST	
Asymmetry	✔
Atypical network	✔
Blue-white structures	✔
Total score	3

Figure 10   Melanoma

This lesion is a straightforward case of melanoma. The diagnostic criteria are striking, obvious asymmetry of color and structure, a markedly atypical pigment network (arrows) and blue-white structures (circle).

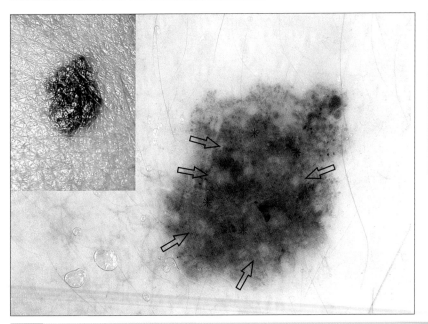

3-POINT CHECKLIST

Asymmetry	☑
Atypical network	☐
Blue-white structures	☐
Total score	1

Figure 11 Nevus
The clinical ABCDs could lead you astray with this banal nevus. There is asymmetry, but there is also a typical pigment network and blue-white structures are absent.

3-POINT CHECKLIST

Asymmetry	☑
Atypical network	☐
Blue-white structures	☑
Total score	2

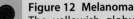

Figure 12 Melanoma
The yellowish globules seen here are not the multiple milia-like cysts of a seborrheic keratosis. They are the ostia of appendages as seen only on head and neck lesions (arrows). There is slight asymmetry of color and structure and no pigment network is observed; however, blue-white structures are seen throughout the lesion (asterisks).

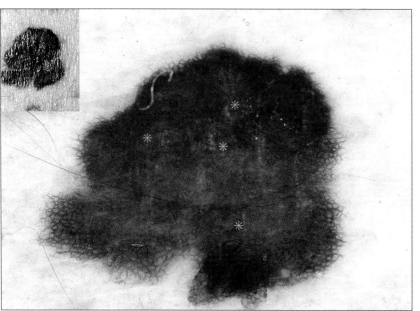

3-POINT CHECKLIST

Asymmetry	✓
Atypical network	✓
Blue-white structures	✓
Total score	3

Figure 13 Melanoma
Clinicians might think that this lesion is nothing to worry about until they examine it with dermoscopy. There is striking asymmetry of color and structure, an atypical pigment network and blue-white structures (asterisks) cover most of the lesion.

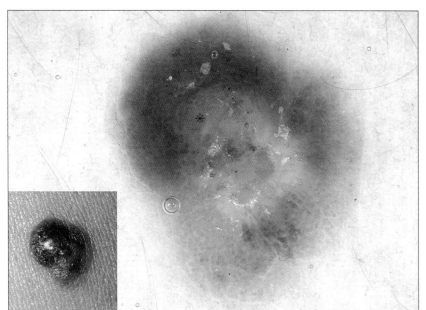

3-POINT CHECKLIST

Asymmetry	✓
Atypical network	☐
Blue-white structures	✓
Total score	2

Figure 14 Melanoma
The blue-white color of regression (asterisk) is the first clue to the seriousness of this lesion. Color and structure are clearly asymmetrical. A pigment network is absent and there are well-developed blue-white structures.

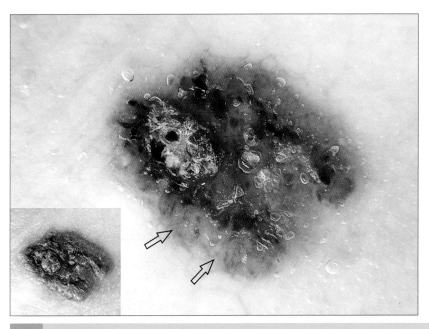

3-POINT CHECKLIST

Asymmetry	✔
Atypical network	
Blue-white structures	✔
Total score	2

Figure 15 Basal cell carcinoma

This lesion is so bizarre-looking that you should excise it as soon as possible. Two positive features of the checklist are clearly present – asymmetry and blue-white structures (arrows). There is no pigment network.

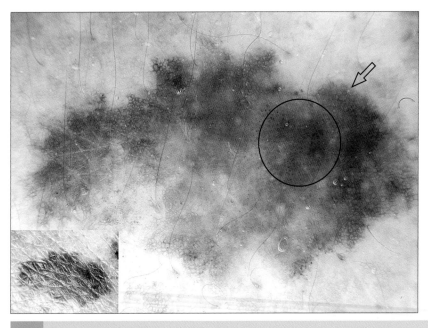

3-POINT CHECKLIST

Asymmetry	✔
Atypical network	✔
Blue-white structures	✔
Total score	3

Figure 16 Melanoma

Asymmetry is unmistakably present in this lesion, but whether the pigment network is atypical in the right upper corner (arrow) is debatable. Blue-white structures (circle) are clearly seen. There is no doubt that it should be excised.

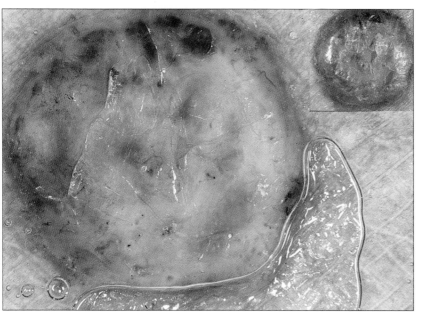

3-POINT CHECKLIST

Asymmetry	✓
Atypical network	☐
Blue-white structures	✓
Total score	2

Figure 17 Basal cell carcinoma

Only two diagnoses are possible for this lesion – hypomelanotic melanoma or hypopigmented basal cell carcinoma. There is asymmetry of color and structure and blue-white structures are found throughout. No pigment network is seen. Because two of the three criteria from the 3-point checklist are present the lesion should be excised.

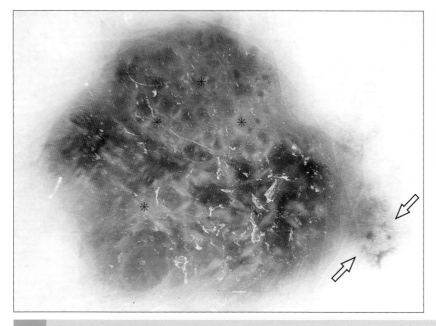

3-POINT CHECKLIST

Asymmetry	✓
Atypical network	☐
Blue-white structures	✓
Total score	2

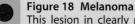

Figure 18 Melanoma

This lesion in clearly not benign. Is it, however, a basal cell carcinoma or melanoma? Once again, there is significant asymmetry of color and structure with prominent blue-white structures (asterisks). It is difficult to decide whether a pigment network is present or not (arrows).

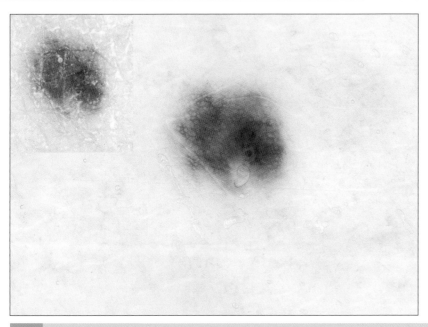

Figure 19 Nevus
This stereotypical benign nevus is commonly seen when performing dermoscopy. The blotch of dark brown color is not significant. Although there is slight asymmetry of color and structure, the lesion is characterized by a typical pigment network and no clearcut blue-white structures are seen.

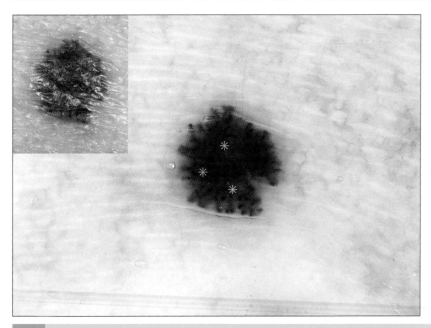

Figure 20 Nevus
The pattern of criteria shown here is most often seen with a Spitz nevus, but the differential diagnosis should include Clark (dysplastic) nevus and melanoma. There is slight asymmetry of color and structure. A pigment network is absent, with blue-white structures (asterisks). The checklist will not work for all lesions and it is important to take into account the history and age of the patient when deciding what to do.

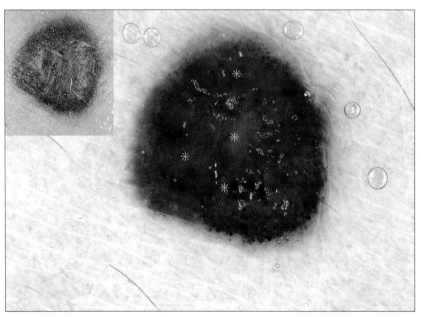

3-POINT CHECKLIST	
Asymmetry	☐
Atypical network	✔
Blue-white structures	✔
Total score	2

Figure 21 Nevus
Another Spitz-nevus-like pattern is demonstrated in this lesion, this time with an atypical pigment network (arrows) and blue-white structures.

3-POINT CHECKLIST	
Asymmetry	✔
Atypical network	☐
Blue-white structures	✔
Total score	2

Figure 22 Melanoma
This banal clinical lesion has a strikingly worrisome dermoscopic appearance, with asymmetry of color and structure. No pigment network is present, but blue-white structures are seen throughout the lesion (asterisks).

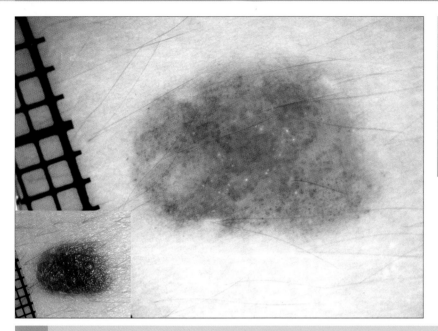

3-POINT CHECKLIST

Asymmetry	✔
Atypical network	☐
Blue-white structures	☐
Total score	1

Figure 23 Nevus
This lesion is benign. Compare it with the other lesions shown in this chapter with more obvious asymmetry of color and structure, an atypical pigment network and blue-white structures. There is slight asymmetry of color and structure, although 100% symmetry is never found in nature. No pigment network or blue-white structures are seen.

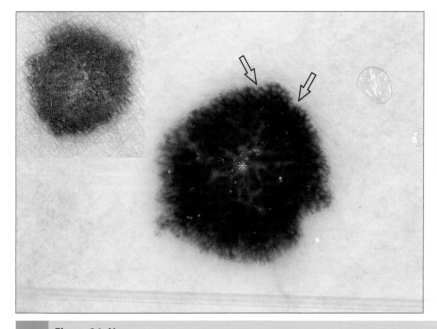

3-POINT CHECKLIST

Asymmetry	✔
Atypical network	✔
Blue-white structures	✔
Total score	3

Figure 24 Nevus
All criteria of the 3-point checklist are present in this lesion, which should therefore be excised. There is asymmetry and an atypical pigment network at the borders (arrows). Blue-white structures are seen in the center of the lesion (asterisk).

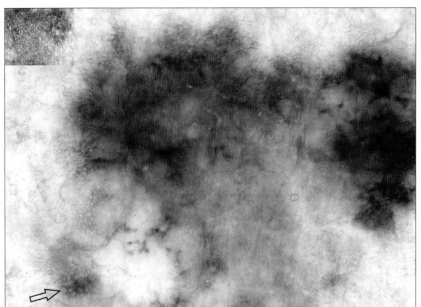

3-POINT CHECKLIST	
Asymmetry	✓
Atypical network	✓
Blue-white structures	✓
Total score	3

Figure 25 Melanoma

This could be a melanoma because of the striking asymmetry of color and structure, and the presence of diffuse blue-white structures throughout the lesion. Several foci of atypical pigment network are also present (arrow).

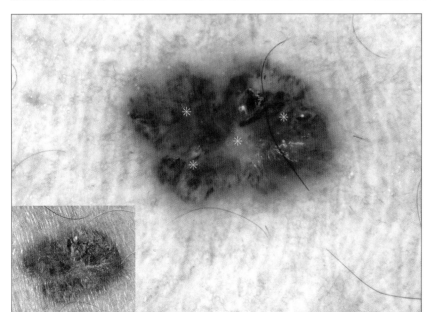

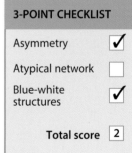

3-POINT CHECKLIST	
Asymmetry	✓
Atypical network	
Blue-white structures	✓
Total score	2

Figure 26 Basal cell carcinoma

There is no doubt that this pigmented neoplasm displays two criteria of the 3-point checklist. Note the striking asymmetry. No pigment network is seen, but several blue-white structures are present (asterisks).

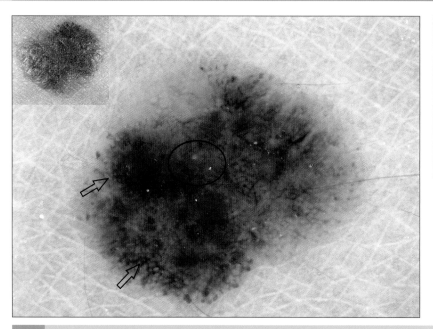

3-POINT CHECKLIST

Asymmetry	✓
Atypical network	✓
Blue-white structures	✓
Total score	3

Figure 27 Melanoma
All three checklist criteria are clearly seen in this lesion. There is significant asymmetry of color and structure with a well-developed atypical pigment network (arrows) and blue-white structures (circle).

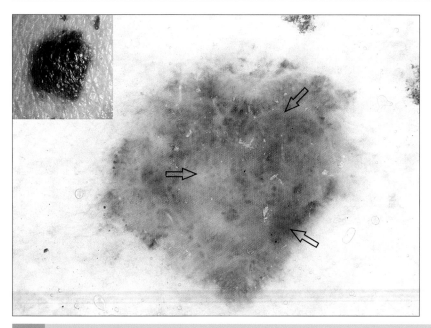

3-POINT CHECKLIST

Asymmetry	✓
Atypical network	
Blue-white structures	✓
Total score	2

Figure 28 Melanoma
Significant asymmetry of color and structure is created by blue-white structures (arrows), which occupy most of the lesion. An atypical pigment network is not seen.

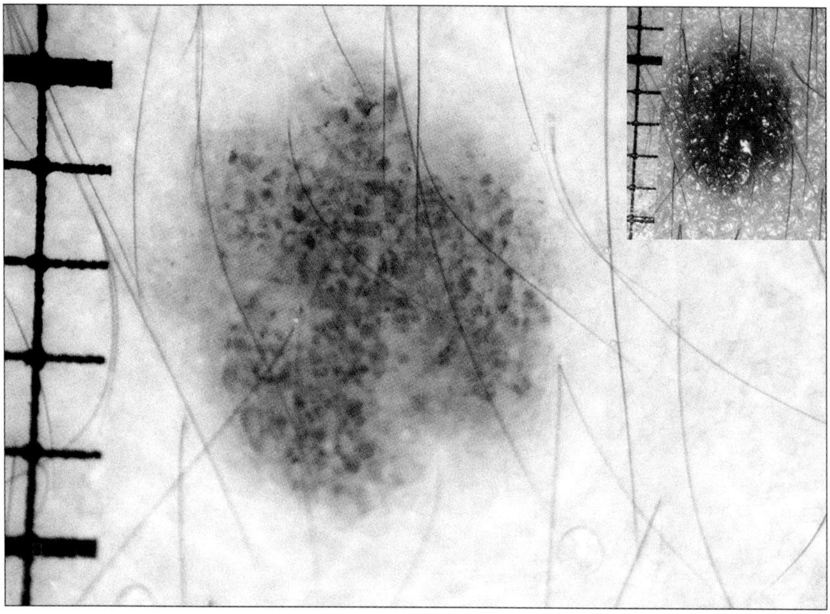

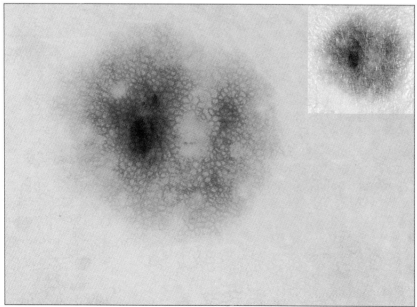

3-POINT CHECKLIST

Asymmetry	✓
Atypical network	☐
Blue-white structures	☐
Total score	1

Figure 29 Nevus

Only one of the checklist criteria is present in this lesion, so this lesion is benign. The lower half of the lesion does not mirror the upper half, thereby displaying subtle asymmetry. No pigment network or blue-white structures are seen.

3-POINT CHECKLIST

Asymmetry	✓
Atypical network	☐
Blue-white structures	☐
Total score	1

Figure 30 Nevus

The presence of a single criterion from the checklist is usually not sufficient to diagnose malignancy. Note the asymmetry of color and structure – the left side of the lesion is not a mirror image of the right side. An atypical pigment network and blue-white structures are absent.

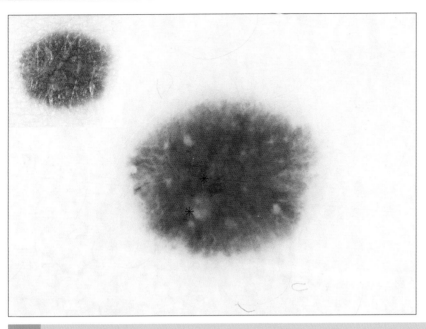

3-POINT CHECKLIST	
Asymmetry	☐
Atypical network	☐
Blue-white structures	✓
Total score	1

Figure 31 Nevus
This is a difficult lesion to interpret. Although only one criterion of the 3-point checklist is present the overall appearance may raise some suspicion that it could be a melanoma. The lesion is symmetrical and there is no pigment network. In the center, blue-white structures are so slight that they might be difficult to detect (asterisks).

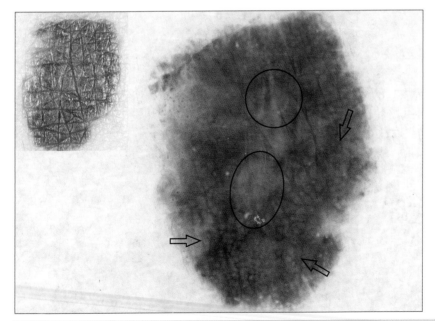

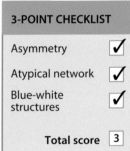

3-POINT CHECKLIST	
Asymmetry	✓
Atypical network	✓
Blue-white structures	✓
Total score	3

Figure 32 Melanoma
All criteria of the 3-point checklist are present, underlining the impression that this lesion is a melanoma. Although the contour is symmetrical, there is asymmetry of color and structure within. A clearcut thickened pigment network (arrows) is present, with small foci of blue-white structures (circles) in the center of the lesion. This early melanoma might go undiagnosed if dermoscopy is not used.

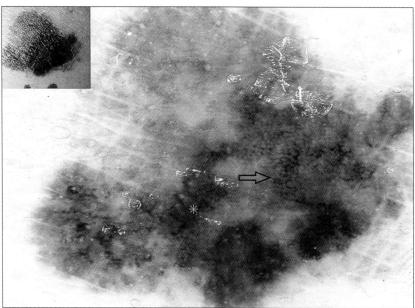

3-POINT CHECKLIST	
Asymmetry	✓
Atypical network	✓
Blue-white structures	✓
Total score	3

Figure 33 Melanoma
Once again, all three features of the checklist are clearly present and even a novice dermoscopist should immediately suspect a melanoma. There is striking asymmetry of color and structure with zones displaying an atypical pigment network (arrow). There are also clearcut areas with blue-white structures (asterisk).

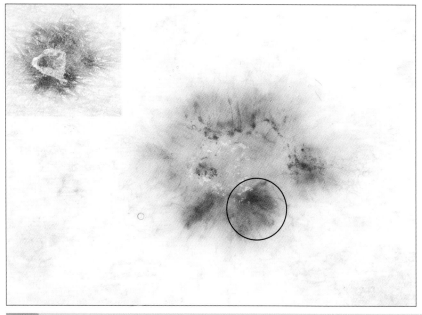

3-POINT CHECKLIST	
Asymmetry	✓
Atypical network	☐
Blue-white structures	✓
Total score	2

Figure 34 Basal cell carcinoma
The lower half of this lesion is not a mirror image of the upper half, and the right side is not a mirror image of the left side; therefore, this is an asymmetrical lesion. No pigment network is identified, but there are numerous blue-white structures seen throughout (circle). Remember, when two criteria are identified the lesion should be excised.

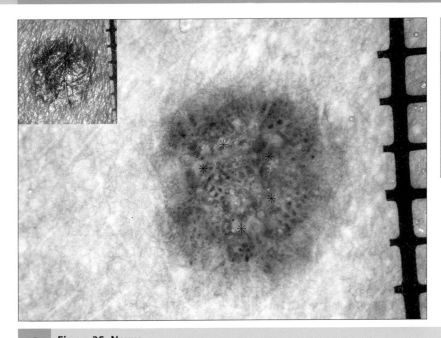

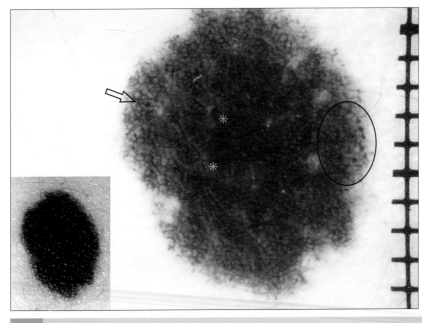

3-POINT CHECKLIST	
Asymmetry	✓
Atypical network	
Blue-white structures	✓
Total score	2

Figure 35 Nevus
Despite the significant asymmetry of color and structure this lesion is benign. There is no hint of a pigment network, but blue-white structures are present (asterisks). With a score of 2, excise this lesion or show it to a more experienced dermoscopist.

3-POINT CHECKLIST	
Asymmetry	✓
Atypical network	✓
Blue-white structures	✓
Total score	3

Figure 36 Nevus
This is a difficult lesion to diagnose because all three features are very subtle. There is an atypical pigment network on the left side (arrow) and globules (circle) on the right side; it is therefore an asymmetrical lesion. Blue-white structures (asterisks) can also be seen throughout.

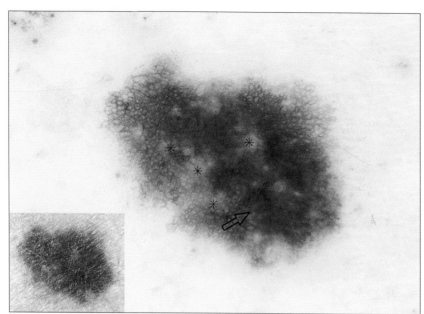

3-POINT CHECKLIST	
Asymmetry	☑
Atypical network	☐
Blue-white structures	☑
Total score	2

Figure 37 Nevus

This is a strikingly asymmetrical lesion but with a typical pigment network. Several subtle foci of blue-white structures are seen (arrow). With two of three checklist criteria present, this lesion should be excised. Do not confuse the multifocal hypopigmentation (asterisks) with the white color that can be seen in blue-white structures.

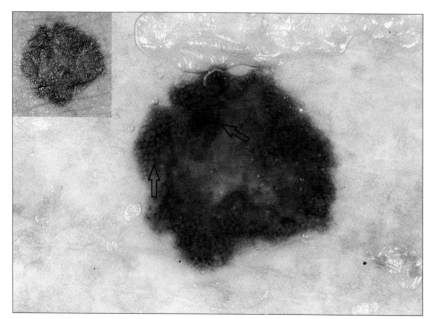
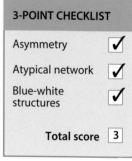

3-POINT CHECKLIST	
Asymmetry	☑
Atypical network	☑
Blue-white structures	☑
Total score	3

Figure 38 Melanoma

Thin melanomas commonly exhibit all three checklist criteria, as demonstrated by this example. There is asymmetry of color and structure with a few foci (arrows) of an atypical pigment network. In the center an area of blue-white structures is also seen. The dermoscopic differential diagnosis includes severely dysplastic nevus and in-situ melanoma with regression.

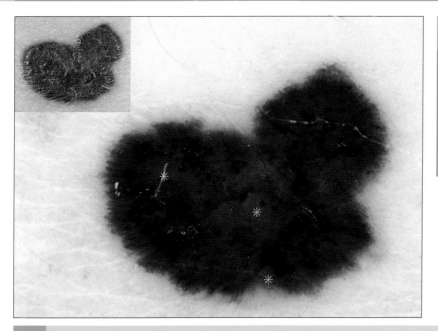

3-POINT CHECKLIST

Asymmetry	☑
Atypical network	☐
Blue-white structures	☑
Total score	2

Figure 39 Melanoma
This dark lesion is a cause for concern. Note the striking asymmetry and multiple blue-white structures varying in size and shape throughout the lesion (asterisks). With two out of three well-developed criteria present, this melanoma will not be misdiagnosed if the 3-point checklist is used.

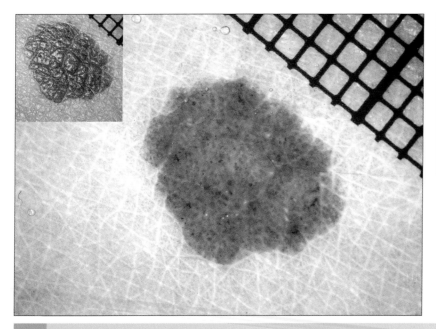

3-POINT CHECKLIST

Asymmetry	☐
Atypical network	☐
Blue-white structures	☐
Total score	0

Figure 40 Nevus
There is an obvious lack of striking criteria in this lesion compared to the melanomas already seen in this chapter. An atypical pigment network and blue-white structures are not seen.

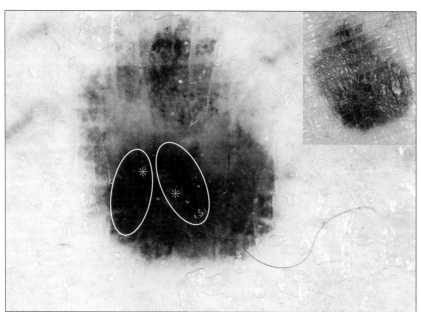

3-POINT CHECKLIST	
Asymmetry	✓
Atypical network	✓
Blue-white structures	✓
Total score	3

Figure 41 Melanoma

This is a clearcut example of a melanoma with a checklist score of 3. There is striking asymmetry of color and structure. Two zones exhibit variations of the morphology of an atypical pigment network (circles), mimicking blotches (structureless hyper-pigmentation). In addition, small foci of blue-white structures can be seen, but with difficulty (asterisks). Always concentrate and focus attention to identify important criteria that might be present in a lesion.

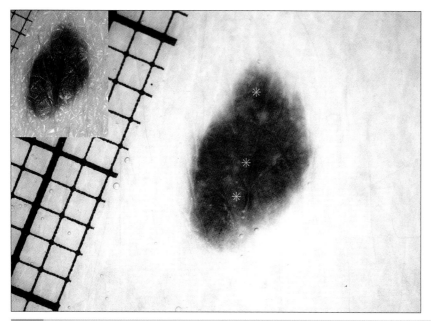

3-POINT CHECKLIST	
Asymmetry	☐
Atypical network	☐
Blue-white structures	✓
Total score	1

Figure 42 Nevus

Numerous foci of blue-white structures are seen throughout (asterisks). An atypical pigment network is not seen. Even though the score is only 1, the dark color and blue-white structures are worrisome. Although it turned out to be a low-risk nevus, it is better to err on the side of safety and remove these borderline lesions. With experience fewer pigmented skin lesions that look like this will be removed.

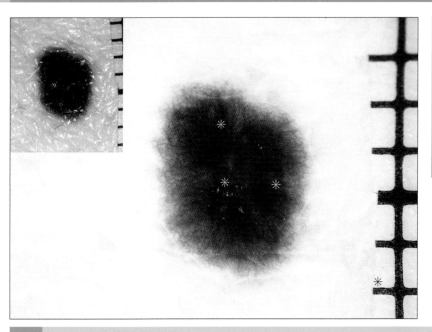

3-POINT CHECKLIST

Asymmetry	☐
Atypical network	☐
Blue-white structures	✓
Total score	1

Figure 43 Nevus

A score of 2 can be achieved for this lesion only if it is considered to be asymmetrical. This image is similar to Figure 42. The pigment network is typical and is therefore not scored. There are, however, numerous foci of blue-white structures (asterisks).

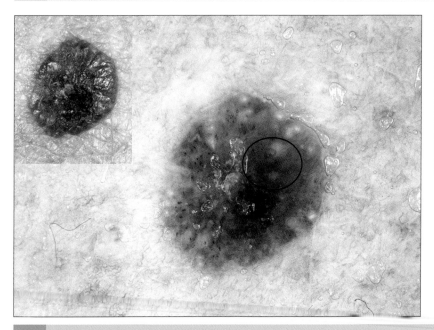

3-POINT CHECKLIST

Asymmetry	✓
Atypical network	☐
Blue-white structures	✓
Total score	2

Figure 44 Seborrheic keratosis

Strictly following the 3-point checklist gives this lesion a score of 2. There is asymmetry of color and structure with a blue-white structure (circle). There is no pigment network. With a score of 2 the novice dermoscopist should remove this lesion, though there will always be exceptions to every rule. With experience clinicians will become confident in diagnosing seborrheic keratosis.

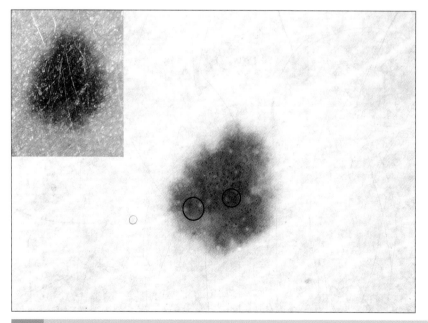

3-POINT CHECKLIST	
Asymmetry	☐
Atypical network	☐
Blue-white structures	☑
Total score	1

Figure 45 Nevus

This lesion has a 3-point checklist score of 1. It is symmetrical and there is no pigment network. Blue-white structures (asterisks), in this instance bony white, are clearly visible. This example can be a potential pitfall for the 3-point checklist because nodular basal cell carcinomas can mimic dermal nevi dermoscopically, particularly when the vascular structures are not carefully examined.

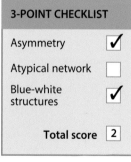

3-POINT CHECKLIST	
Asymmetry	☑
Atypical network	☐
Blue-white structures	☑
Total score	2

Figure 46 Nevus

This is another difficult lesion to diagnose because its checklist score may be 1 or 2. Always remember: if a lesion could be high risk, excise it or follow the patient closely. There is slight but distinct asymmetry of dermoscopic structures but no pigment network. Very subtle hints of blue-white structures (circles) may be seen.

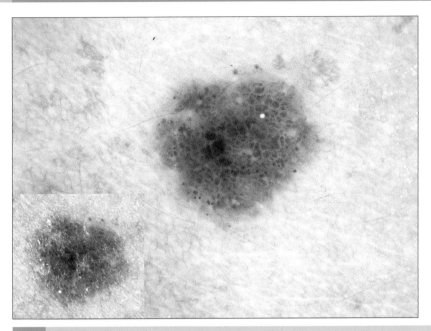

3-POINT CHECKLIST

Asymmetry	✓
Atypical network	☐
Blue-white structures	☐
Total score	1

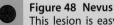

Figure 47 Nevus
The checklist score for this lesion is only 1, with slight asymmetry of color and structure.

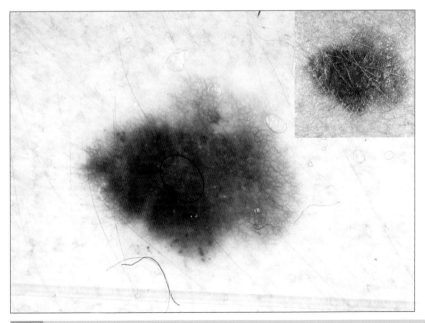

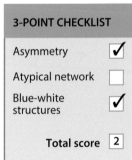

3-POINT CHECKLIST

Asymmetry	✓
Atypical network	☐
Blue-white structures	✓
Total score	2

Figure 48 Nevus
This lesion is easy to handle from a management point of view because two of the three checklist criteria are present, so it should be excised. There is noticeable asymmetry of color and structure and blue-white structures (circle) are found in the left half of the lesion. The pigment network, however, is not atypical.

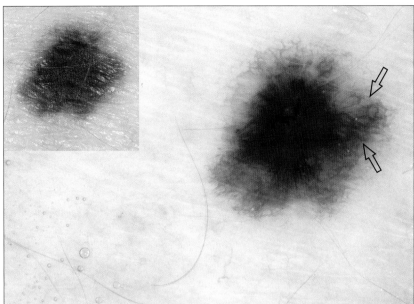

3-POINT CHECKLIST	
Asymmetry	✓
Atypical network	✓
Blue-white structures	☐
Total score	2

Figure 49 Nevus

This dermoscopic image is worrisome, showing two of the three checklist criteria. There is asymmetry of color and structure and an atypical thickened and branched pigment network (arrows). The novice should excise a lesion with this dermoscopic appearance although the pathology report might not be high risk.

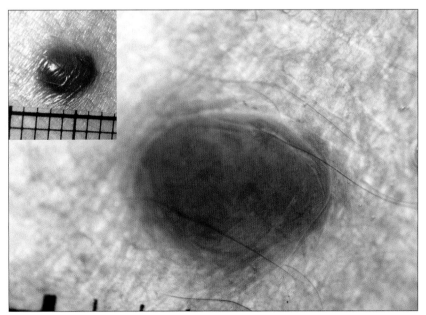

3-POINT CHECKLIST	
Asymmetry	☐
Atypical network	☐
Blue-white structures	✓
Total score	1

Figure 50 Nevus

This is a blue nevus for which the checklist score is obviously 1. This lesion is symmetrical without a pigment network, but blue-white structures are seen homogeneously throughout the lesion. The dermoscopic appearance of blue nevi is unique, but always be cautious when making the diagnosis because rarely nodular melanoma and cutaneous metastatic melanoma mimic a blue nevus.

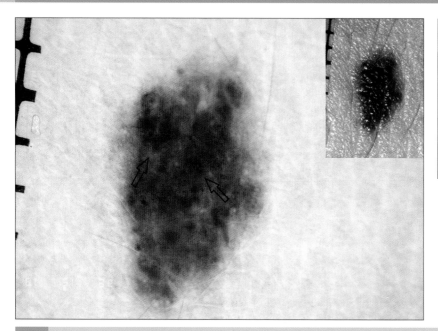

3-POINT CHECKLIST	
Asymmetry	✔
Atypical network	
Blue-white structures	✔
Total score	2

Figure 51 Nevus

Again, the management of this lesion after evaluating it with the 3-point checklist is straightforward. With a score of 2, this could be a high-risk lesion. There is striking asymmetry of color and structure. Foci of blue-white structures (arrows) are observed mainly in the upper half of the lesion. No pigment network is seen. The discordance between the positive 3-point checklist score and the banal pathology can be explained by the uneven pigmentation of nests of melanocytes at the level of the junction and papillary dermis.

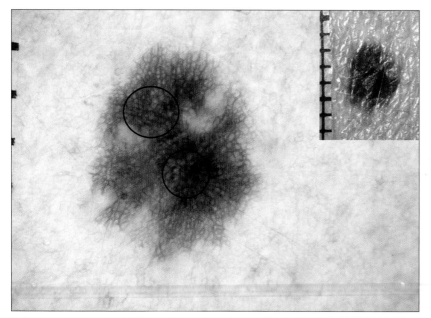

3-POINT CHECKLIST	
Asymmetry	✔
Atypical network	✔
Blue-white structures	
Total score	2

Figure 52 Nevus

The checklist score for this lesion is 2. There is slight asymmetry of structure with foci of atypical pigment network (circles).

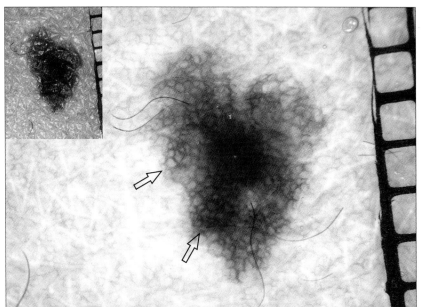

3-POINT CHECKLIST

Asymmetry	☑
Atypical network	☑
Blue-white structures	☐
Total score	2

Figure 53 Nevus
This lesion also has a checklist score of 2. This example shows the limitations of the 3-point checklist. There is asymmetry because the lower half does not mirror the upper half. Also note that the pigment network is atypical (arrows). Blue-white structures are not observed.

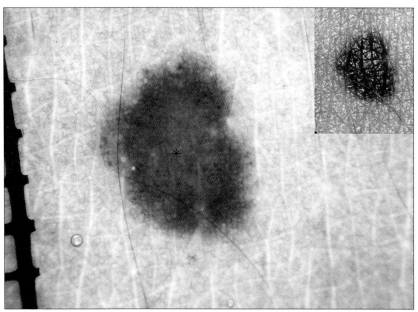

3-POINT CHECKLIST

Asymmetry	☑
Atypical network	☐
Blue-white structures	☐
Total score	1

Figure 54 Nevus
This lesion is asymmetrical because the left side is not a mirror image of the right side. The line segments of the pigment network are not thick, dark or branched; therefore, it is not atypical. Do not confuse the central hypopigmentation (asterisk) with blue-white structures.

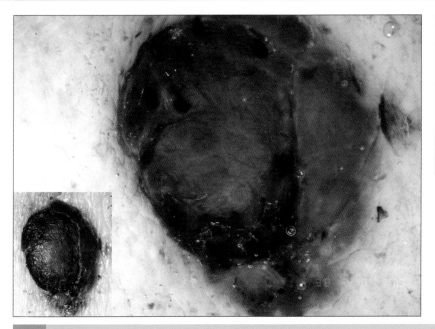

3-POINT CHECKLIST

Asymmetry	✓
Atypical network	☐
Blue-white structures	✓
Total score	2

Figure 55 Melanoma

There are two strikingly positive features present here – asymmetry and blue-white structures. Because the lesion is nodular it should be excised. Clearcut asymmetry of color and structure and conspicuous blue-white structures are seen throughout the lesion. No pigment network is seen, not even at the periphery. There is commonly a complete lack of pigment network in thick nodular melanomas. This lesion was diagnosed clinically as seborrheic keratosis. It was lucky for the patient that its dermoscopic appearance was suspicious enough to warrant excision.

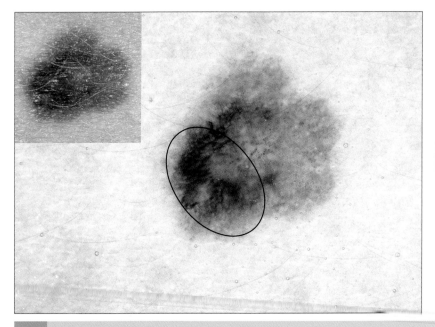

3-POINT CHECKLIST

Asymmetry	✓
Atypical network	✓
Blue-white structures	☐
Total score	2

Figure 56 Nevus

The atypical pigment network (circle) in this asymmetrical lesion is worrisome and the lesion should be excised. No blue-white structures are seen. Although the histology was benign, this dermoscopic picture might also be seen in in-situ melanoma.

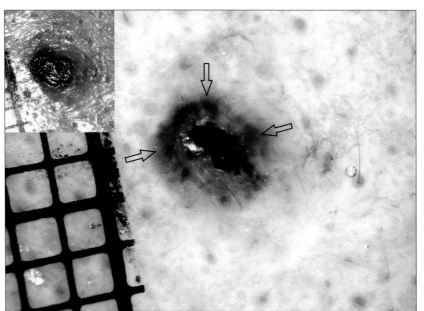
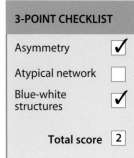

3-POINT CHECKLIST	
Asymmetry	✓
Atypical network	☐
Blue-white structures	✓
Total score	2

Figure 57 Basal cell carcinoma
The checklist score for this lesion is 2; because it is nodular, excision is recommended. Note the asymmetry of color and structure and several blue-white structures (arrows). No pigment network can be identified.

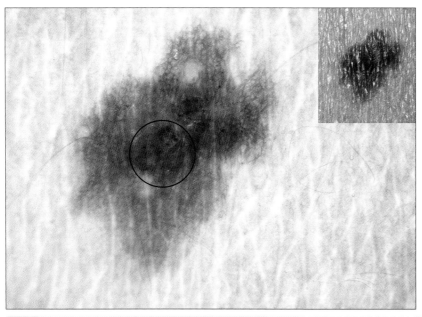

3-POINT CHECKLIST	
Asymmetry	✓
Atypical network	☐
Blue-white structures	✓
Total score	2

Figure 58 Nevus
Two of the 3-point checklist criteria are present. Striking asymmetry of color and structure and a few blue-white structures (circle) are seen.

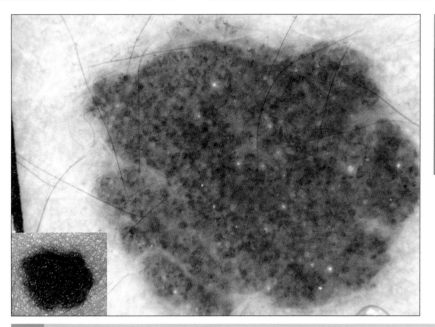

3-POINT CHECKLIST

Asymmetry	☐
Atypical network	☐
Blue-white structures	☐
Total score	0

Figure 59 Nevus
The checklist score for this lesion is zero.

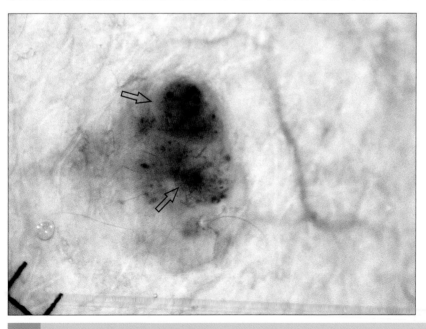

3-POINT CHECKLIST

Asymmetry	✔
Atypical network	☐
Blue-white structures	✔
Total score	2

Figure 60 Basal cell carcinoma
This nodular lesion scores 2, so should be excised.
There is asymmetry of color and structure. Note the
few blue-white structures (arrows) in the absence of
a pigment network.

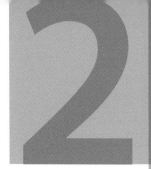

Pattern Analysis

Dermoscopic criteria for specific diagnoses

Dermoscopic analysis of pigmented skin lesions is based on four algorithms:

- pattern analysis;
- the ABCD rule;
- Menzies' 11-point checklist; and
- the 7-point checklist

The common denominator of all these diagnostic algorithms is the identification and analysis of dermoscopic criteria found in the lesions. The majority of the dermatologists who participated in the second consensus meeting were proponents of pattern analysis. The basic principle is that pigmented skin lesions are characterized by global patterns and combinations of local criteria.

FIVE GLOBAL DERMOSCOPIC PATTERNS FOR MELANOCYTIC NEVI

RETICULAR PATTERN

The reticular pattern is the most common global pattern in melanocytic lesions. It is characterized by a pigment network covering most parts of a lesion. The pigment network appears as a grid of line segments (honeycomb-like) in different shades of black, brown or gray. Modifications of the pigment network vary with changes in the biologic behavior of melanocytic skin lesions, and these variations therefore merit special attention.

GLOBULAR PATTERN

Variously-sized, round-to-oval brown structures fill these melanocytic lesions. This pattern can be found in congenital and acquired melanocytic and Clark (dysplastic) nevi.

HOMOGENEOUS PATTERN

This pattern is characterized by a diffuse, uniform, structureless color filling most of the lesion. Colors include black, brown, gray, blue, white or red. A predominantly bluish color is the morphologic hallmark of blue nevi.

STARBURST PATTERN

The starburst pattern is characterized by the presence of pigmented streaks and/or dots and globules in a radial arrangement at the periphery of a melanocytic lesion. This pattern is the stereotypical morphology in Spitz nevi.

NON-SPECIFIC PATTERN

In some instances a melanocytic lesion cannot be categorized into one of the global patterns listed above and is therefore categorized as having a 'non-specific pattern'. A non-specific pattern may be found in melanoma.

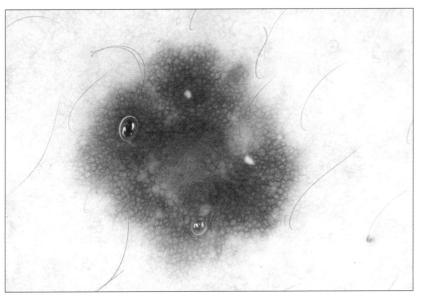

FIVE GLOBAL PATTERNS FOR MELANOCYTIC NEVI

Reticular pattern	✔
Globular pattern	☐
Homogeneous pattern	☐
Starburst pattern	☐
Non-specific pattern	☐

Figure 61 Nevus

The reticular type is probably the most common dermoscopic feature of a flat acquired melanocytic nevus. It is characterized by a typical pigment network that fades out at the periphery. There are also a few small islands of hypopigmentation – a common finding in benign nevi. The histopathologic distinction between a junctional nevus and a compound nevus is commonly given, but the distinction cannot always be made dermoscopically. Moreover, it is clinically irrelevant.

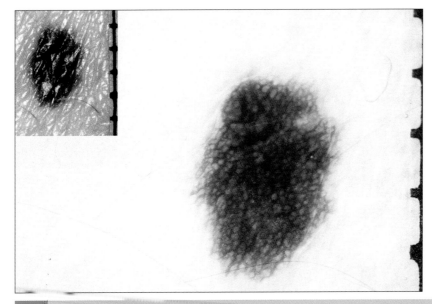

FIVE GLOBAL PATTERNS FOR MELANOCYTIC NEVI

Reticular pattern	✔
Globular pattern	☐
Homogeneous pattern	☐
Starburst pattern	☐
Non-specific pattern	☐

Figure 62 Nevus

Here is another example of the morphology seen with the reticular type of banal nevus. The quality of the typical pigment network demonstrates darker and thicker lines. The benign nature of this lesion is emphasized by the fading out at the periphery of the pigment network.

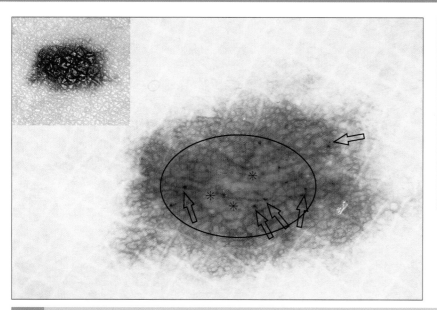

FIVE GLOBAL PATTERNS FOR MELANOCYTIC NEVI

Reticular pattern	✔
Globular pattern	☐
Homogeneous pattern	☐
Starburst pattern	☐
Non-specific pattern	☐

Figure 63 Nevus

This is a reticular-type lesion with a few dots. In the center of the lesion the lines of the pigment network are slightly thicker and more heavily pigmented (circle). In addition, there are a few dark-brown dots (arrows) and a hint of a blue-white structure (asterisks). Again, note the fading out of the pigment network along the entire periphery of the lesion representing an important clue that this is a benign melanocytic lesion. This can also be called a Clark, dysplastic or atypical nevus; it is not a melanoma.

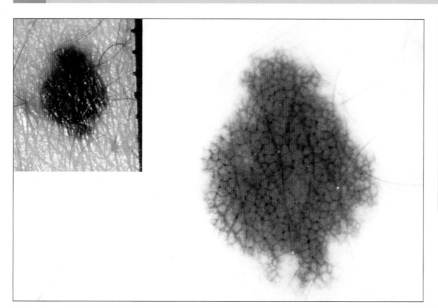

FIVE GLOBAL PATTERNS FOR MELANOCYTIC NEVI

Reticular pattern	✔
Globular pattern	☐
Homogeneous pattern	☐
Starburst pattern	☐
Non-specific pattern	☐

Figure 64 Nevus

This lesion is characterized by a typical pigment network and numerous dots, which are situated on the crossing points of the network lines. In the background, diffuse blue-white structures can be seen covering most of the lesion. Histopatho-logically, the diffuse blue-white structures represent a dense infiltrate of melanophages in the papillary dermis. The differentiation between a junctional and a compound nevus is not possible dermoscopi-cally.

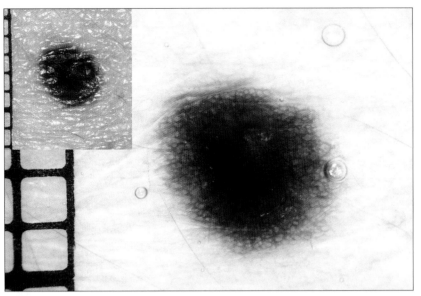

FIVE GLOBAL PATTERNS FOR MELANOCYTIC NEVI

Reticular pattern	✔
Globular pattern	☐
Homogeneous pattern	✔
Starburst pattern	☐
Non-specific pattern	☐

Figure 65 Nevus

A reticular–homogeneous pattern, as seen here, can be seen in banal nevi. In the center there is homogeneous black pigmentation (black lamella) and at the periphery there is an annular distribution of a typical pigment network. Once again, the pigment network fades at the periphery – a sign of a benign nature. If this was a solitary lesion, in-situ melanoma would be the differential diagnosis. Most people with this dermoscopic appearance have multiple similar-appearing nevi, favoring low-risk pathology. Tape stripping can peel away the black lamella and allows one to see whether there are any underlying typical or atypical structures.

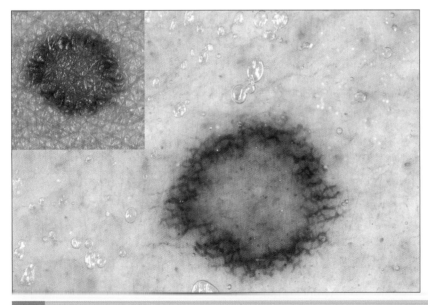

FIVE GLOBAL PATTERNS FOR MELANOCYTIC NEVI

Reticular pattern	✔
Globular pattern	☐
Homogeneous pattern	✔
Starburst pattern	☐
Non-specific pattern	☐

Figure 66 Nevus

The unusual type of reticular–homogeneous pattern seen here is more often found in younger pediatric patients. In the center of the lesion there is homogeneous hypopigmentation (not to be confused with the bony–milky white color of regression), and this is surrounded by a small rim of pigment network. The lines of the pigment network are thickened and the meshes are slightly irregular. The overall architecture of the network, however, is symmetrical and regular.

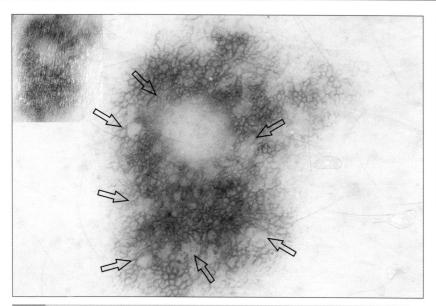

FIVE GLOBAL PATTERNS FOR MELANOCYTIC NEVI

Reticular pattern	✔
Globular pattern	☐
Homogeneous pattern	✔
Starburst pattern	☐
Non-specific pattern	☐

Figure 67 Nevus

A stereotypical reticular pattern is seen here. The pigment network is typical, but unevenly distributed and fades out at the periphery. In addition, there are hypopigmented areas throughout the lesion (arrows). This nevus does not reveal criteria used to diagnose melanoma (melanoma-specific criteria). Because of the uneven distribution of the pigment network and variations in the shades of brown, the novice dermoscopist should consider excision or close dermoscopic and clinical follow-up.

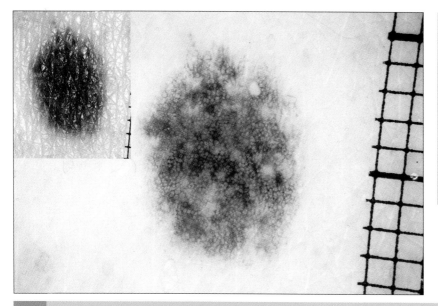

FIVE GLOBAL PATTERNS FOR MELANOCYTIC NEVI

Reticular pattern	✔
Globular pattern	☐
Homogeneous pattern	☐
Starburst pattern	☐
Non-specific pattern	☐

Figure 68 Nevus

The patchy reticular pattern shown here is associated with an uneven distribution of a typical pigment network. The intensity of pigmentation of the lines alternates, giving this pigment network a patchy appearance, and is similar to Figure 67. The general principle to remember is that any unevenness of relatively regular-appearing criteria is a minor cause for concern.

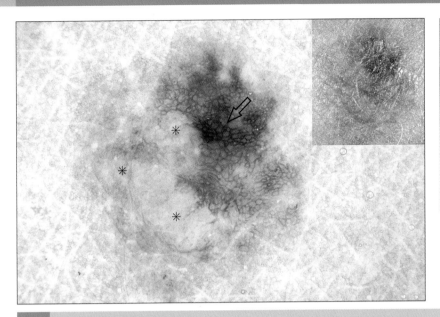

FIVE GLOBAL PATTERNS FOR MELANOCYTIC NEVI	
Reticular pattern	✔
Globular pattern	☐
Homogeneous pattern	✔
Starburst pattern	☐
Non-specific pattern	☐

Figure 69 Nevus

This nevus shows a variation of reticular-pattern morphology. Note the zone of atypical pigment network in the upper part of this lesion characterized by darker pigmentation and thickening of the line segments (arrow). The large area of hypopigmentation (asterisks) is not an area of regression that would be seen in melanoma. It is not bony–milky white. If in doubt, cut it out.

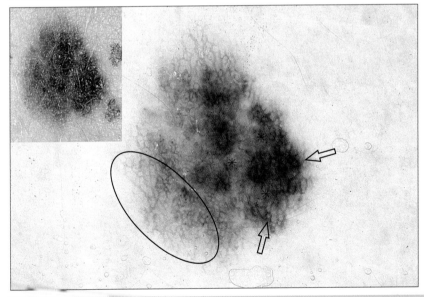

FIVE GLOBAL PATTERNS FOR MELANOCYTIC NEVI	
Reticular pattern	✔
Globular pattern	☐
Homogeneous pattern	☐
Starburst pattern	☐
Non-specific pattern	☐

Figure 70 Nevus

This dermoscopic picture is very worrying. The reticular pattern with eccentric hyperpigmentation dermoscopically simulates in-situ melanoma arising in a pre-existing nevus. The right half of this lesion is characterized by an atypical pigment network (arrows) intermingled with blue-white structures (asterisks). On the left side there is a bland pigment network (circle) characteristic of a benign nevus. Do not hesitate to excise a lesion that looks like this as soon as possible. The final histopathologic diagnosis is in-situ melanoma within a pre-existing nevus in 10% of similar-appearing lesions. In this case, the diagnosis was Clark (dysplastic) nevus, compound type.

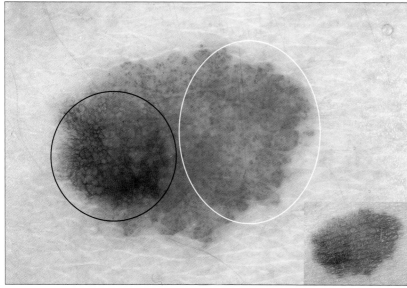

FIVE GLOBAL PATTERNS FOR MELANOCYTIC NEVI	
Reticular pattern	✔
Globular pattern	☐
Homogeneous pattern	☐
Starburst pattern	☐
Non-specific pattern	☐

Figure 71 Nevus

This nevus also shows eccentric hyperpigmentation and simulates melanoma in association with a pre-existing nevus. It is characterized by two different areas: the upper right area has a typical (circle) pigment network; the lower left side is characterized by dark-brown and black pigmentation and by several irregular dots and globules (arrows) and hints of a blue-white structure (asterisk). This lesion should undoubtedly be excised because there are melanoma-specific criteria (described later in this chapter): irregular dots and globules, and blue-white structures. Despite the suspicious dermoscopic appearance this lesion turned out to be a Clark (dysplastic) nevus.

FIVE GLOBAL PATTERNS FOR MELANOCYTIC NEVI	
Reticular pattern	✔
Globular pattern	✔
Homogeneous pattern	☐
Starburst pattern	☐
Non-specific pattern	☐

Figure 72 Nevus

The reticular (black circle)–globular (white circle) pattern with eccentric hyperpigmentation shown here once again raises the possibility of a melanoma. The right side of the lesion demonstrates diffuse hypopigmented areas and numerous regular dots and globules. The left side has a definite atypical pigment network (black circle) with thickened, branched line segments. This lesion was excised and histopathologically diagnosed as Clark (dysplastic) nevus, compound type.

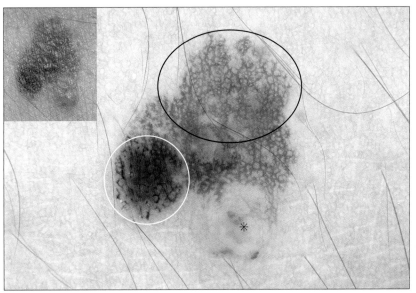

FIVE GLOBAL PATTERNS FOR MELANOCYTIC NEVI

Reticular pattern	✔
Globular pattern	☐
Homogeneous pattern	✔
Starburst pattern	☐
Non-specific pattern	☐

Figure 73 Nevus

Here is another lesion with a reticular pattern and eccentric hyperpigmentation. It is composed of three different areas (multicomponent pattern): a reticular part in the upper half characterized by a slightly thickened but typical pigment network (black circle); a lower part with round hypopigmentation clinically resembling a small papule (asterisk); another small roundish zone with an atypical pigment network in the left corner (white circle). A subtle blue-white structure is also seen in this area. This lesion was excised and histopathologically diagnosed as a Clark (dysplastic) nevus, compound type. Despite the benign diagnosis of all of these cases, eccentric hyperpigmentation should always be a cause for concern.

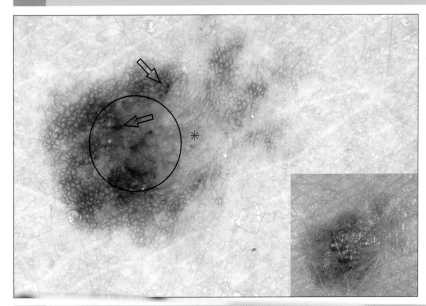

FIVE GLOBAL PATTERNS FOR MELANOCYTIC NEVI

Reticular pattern	✔
Globular pattern	☐
Homogeneous pattern	☐
Starburst pattern	☐
Non-specific pattern	☐

Figure 74 Nevus

This lesion has enough pigment network to qualify as having a reticular pattern. There is a central zone of hypopigmentation (asterisk) and a few irregular dots and globules (arrows). The pigment network has different qualities throughout the lesion. It is thickened in the center and thins out along the periphery. The blue-white structure (circle) is an important sign and indicates that this is potentially a high-risk lesion. Histopathologically, this was diagnosed as a compound type of Clark (dysplastic) nevus. Novice dermoscopists should not hesitate to excise lesions that look like this.

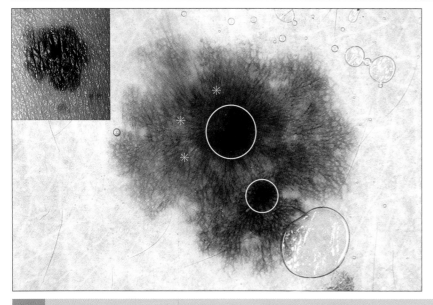

FIVE GLOBAL
PATTERNS FOR
MELANOCYTIC NEVI

Reticular pattern	✔
Globular pattern	☐
Homogeneous pattern	☐
Starburst pattern	☐
Non-specific pattern	☐

Figure 75 Nevus

This is another example of a reticular pattern, with a slightly atypical pigment network that thins out along the periphery. In the center there is hyperpigmentation (circle) with a few irregular dots and globules (arrows) and there are subtle blue-white structures (asterisks). These signs are sufficient to warrant excision. In the realm of Clark (dysplastic) nevi it is difficult to determine whether the lesion is low or high risk dermoscopically; therefore the novice is best advised to excise gray zone lesions.

FIVE GLOBAL
PATTERNS FOR
MELANOCYTIC NEVI

Reticular pattern	✔
Globular pattern	☐
Homogeneous pattern	☐
Starburst pattern	☐
Non-specific pattern	☐

Figure 76 Nevus

This lesion has a reticular pattern with central hyperpigmentation. In the center of the lesion there are two irregular black blotches (circles). The larger one is surrounded by blue-white structures (asterisks). The pigment network is atypical because the color varies in intensity and the lines are thickened and branched. Although this lesion is benign, it simulates melanoma and should be excised.

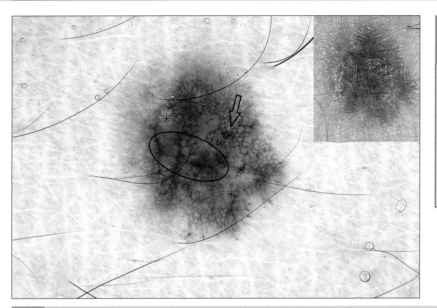

FIVE GLOBAL PATTERNS FOR MELANOCYTIC NEVI

Reticular pattern	✔
Globular pattern	☐
Homogeneous pattern	☐
Starburst pattern	☐
Non-specific pattern	☐

Figure 77 Nevus

This is another example of the variation of morphology with the reticular pattern. The pigment network is mostly typical with a tendency to thin out at the periphery, but there are some areas where it is thickened and branched (arrow). Hypopigmented areas (asterisks) and a few subtle blue-white structures (circle) are also seen. This Clark (dysplastic) nevus simulates in-situ melanoma and should be excised.

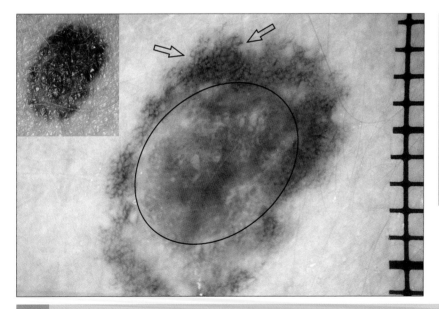

FIVE GLOBAL PATTERNS FOR MELANOCYTIC NEVI

Reticular pattern	✔
Globular pattern	☐
Homogeneous pattern	✔
Starburst pattern	☐
Non-specific pattern	☐

Figure 78 Nevus

This nevus simulates a superficial melanoma and excision is indicated. In the center there are blue-white structures (circle) and an atypical pigment network with an annular distribution is seen at the periphery. In the upper half of the lesion, the pigment network ends abruptly at the border (arrows). This picture warrants a second pathologic opinion because it looks like a melanoma. There is no 'gold standard' from a histopathologic point of view. Experienced dermatopathologists often give a different diagnosis for the same melanocytic lesion. Do not hesitate to get a second opinion.

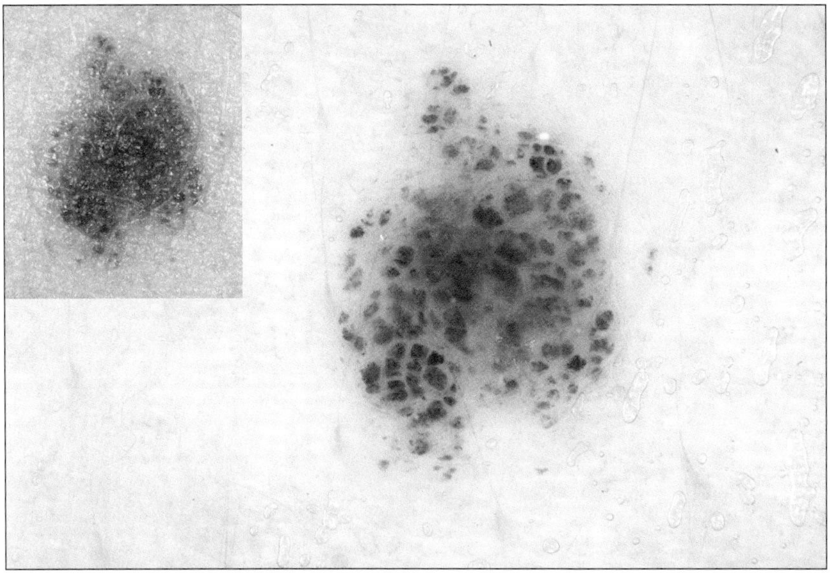

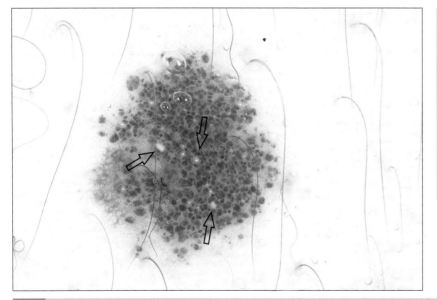

Figure 79 Nevus

This shows a stereotypical globular pattern of a benign nevus. There are numerous dots and globules of similar shape and varying size throughout the lesion. No melanoma-specific dermoscopic criteria are seen. This pattern is most commonly seen in adolescents, but can also be found in adults. The histopathology could be a junctional or compound nevus.

Figure 80 Nevus

This shows one of the many variations of the morphology seen with the globular pattern. The most relevant aspect of this lesion is the even distribution of closely packed, similar-appearing dots and globules. In addition, there are a few milia-like cysts in the center of the lesion (arrows). Milia-like cysts are not seen only in seborrheic keratosis.

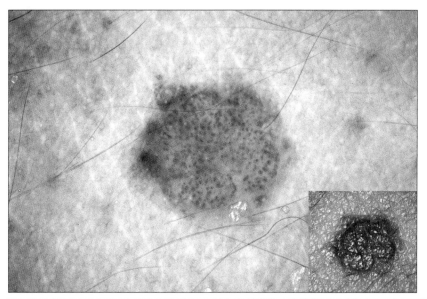

FIVE GLOBAL PATTERNS FOR MELANOCYTIC NEVI

Reticular pattern	☐
Globular pattern	✔
Homogeneous pattern	☐
Starburst pattern	☐
Non-specific pattern	☐

Figure 81 Nevus

This globular pattern shows dots and globules that are not closely packed together, are similar in size and shape, and have a slightly uneven distribution. No melanoma-specific criteria are seen in this banal lesion.

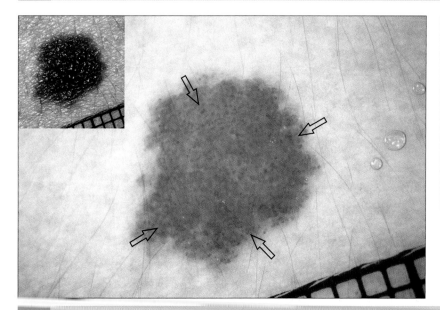

FIVE GLOBAL PATTERNS FOR MELANOCYTIC NEVI

Reticular pattern	☐
Globular pattern	✔
Homogeneous pattern	☐
Starburst pattern	☐
Non-specific pattern	☐

Figure 82 Nevus

Most of this lesion is characterized by homogeneous light-brown pigmentation and subtle dots and globules (arrows).

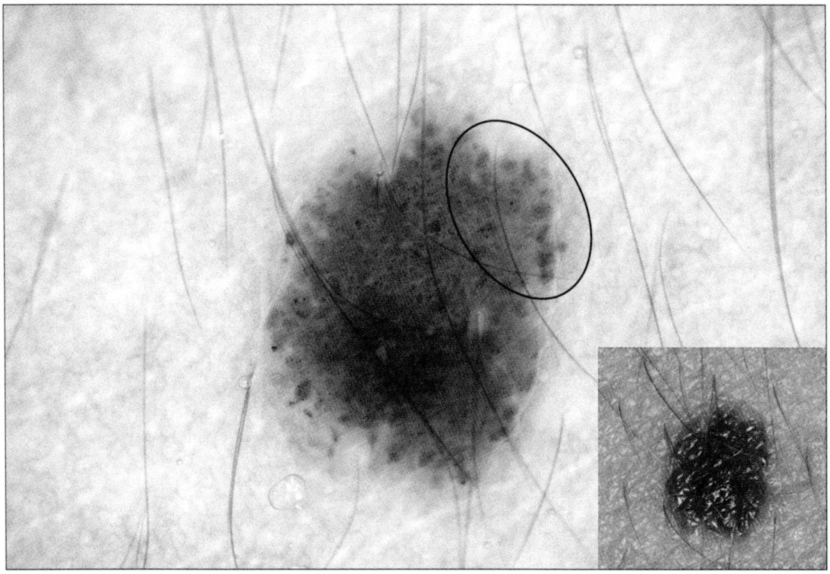

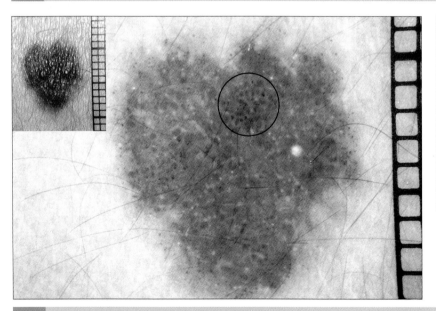

**FIVE GLOBAL
PATTERNS FOR
MELANOCYTIC NEVI**

Reticular pattern	☐
Globular pattern	☑
Homogeneous pattern	☐
Starburst pattern	☐
Non-specific pattern	☐

Figure 83 Nevus
This image shows a more worrisome variation of the globular pattern. Numerous dots and globules are unevenly distributed throughout the lesion (circle) and vary in size and shape.

**FIVE GLOBAL
PATTERNS FOR
MELANOCYTIC NEVI**

Reticular pattern	☐
Globular pattern	☑
Homogeneous pattern	☐
Starburst pattern	☐
Non-specific pattern	☐

Figure 84 Nevus
Here is another globular type of nevus. Numerous light-brown to blue-gray dots and globules, which are of similar size and shape, are distributed regularly throughout the lesion. The only worrisome area is a collection of about 15–20 gray globules (circle), which prompted the excision of this compound type of Clark (dysplastic) nevus. Study lesions carefully to look for subtle yet potentially high-risk criteria.

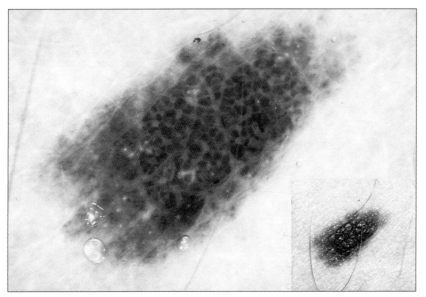

FIVE GLOBAL PATTERNS FOR MELANOCYTIC NEVI

Reticular pattern	☐
Globular pattern	✔
Homogeneous pattern	☐
Starburst pattern	☐
Non-specific pattern	☐

Figure 85 Nevus

This is another stereotypical example of the globular pattern of nevus, in which the globules are very easy to see. In the center of this lesion numerous dark-brown dots and globules with a rectangular shape (cobblestone-like) are present and are surrounded by a rim of brown pigmentation. Dermoscopically this lesion gives the impression of a papillomatous or raised character. Histopathologic examination revealed a compound nevus.

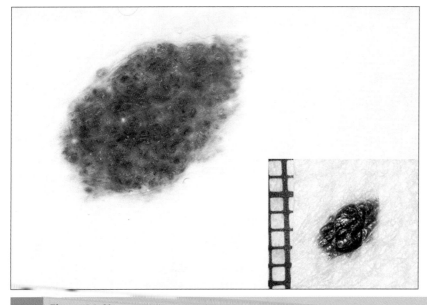

FIVE GLOBAL PATTERNS FOR MELANOCYTIC NEVI

Reticular pattern	☐
Globular pattern	✔
Homogeneous pattern	☐
Starburst pattern	☐
Non-specific pattern	☐

Figure 86 Nevus

The globular pattern seen here is similar to that in Figure 85, yet the globules are not that easy to see. The lesion is composed of closely packed gray dots and globules. No other dermoscopic criteria are observed. The variation of the color might alarm the inexperienced dermoscopist. Remember, if in doubt cut it out. This was a benign nevus. After seeing and excising a few lesions with this dermoscopic appearance, the dermoscopist will feel more comfortable about not excising lesions that look like this.

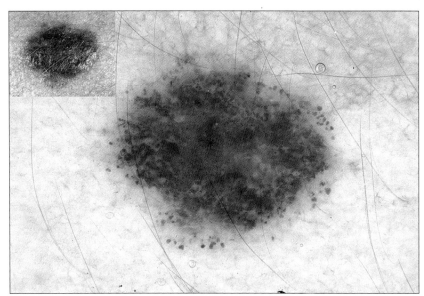

Figure 87 Nevus

This lesion shows another variant of the globular pattern. It contains numerous tiny brown-to-gray dots and globules, which are evenly distributed throughout the lesion. There is a definite blue-white structure (asterisk) in the center. A blue-white structure and diffuse dots and globules is a pattern that can be seen with Spitz nevi. This is spitzoid.

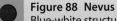

Figure 88 Nevus

Blue-white structures (asterisk) are seen in the center of this globular type of nevus. One important finding is dots and globules along the periphery. This indicates a changing active lesion and can be seen in banal nevi, Clark (dysplastic) nevi and melanomas. Because of the dermoscopic asymmetry and the peripheral rim of dots and globules this lesion was excised. Histopathologically it was a compound type of Clark (dysplastic) nevus. A peripheral rim of dots and globules indicates an actively changing lesion. Beware!

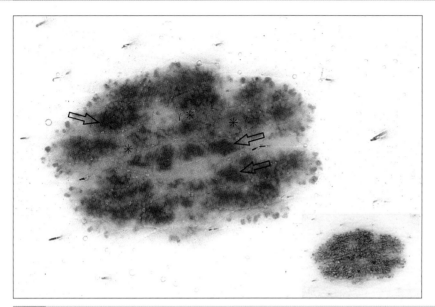

FIVE GLOBAL PATTERNS FOR MELANOCYTIC NEVI

Reticular pattern	☐
Globular pattern	☑
Homogeneous pattern	☐
Starburst pattern	☐
Non-specific pattern	☐

Figure 89 Nevus

This melanocytic proliferation looks high risk, being characterized by a patchy distribution of an otherwise typical pigment network and surrounded by numerous regular dots and globules in an annular distribution at the periphery. In addition, there are a few clearly visible blue-white structures (asterisks) and multiple irregular blotches of pigmentation (arrows). The dermoscopic differential diagnosis includes a high-risk Clark (dysplastic) nevus or melanoma with regression. The final histopathologic diagnosis was a compound type of Clark (dysplastic) nevus.

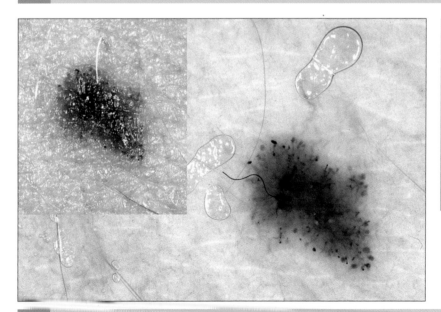

FIVE GLOBAL PATTERNS FOR MELANOCYTIC NEVI

Reticular pattern	☐
Globular pattern	☑
Homogeneous pattern	☐
Starburst pattern	☐
Non-specific pattern	☐

Figure 90 Nevus

Numerous irregularly sized brownish dots and globules are seen throughout this lesion. Although it is very small, the dermoscopic asymmetry is striking. The pinkish color is an important clue that this could be a high-risk lesion. This warrants a second histopathologic opinion because of the benign diagnosis, despite its high-risk appearance.

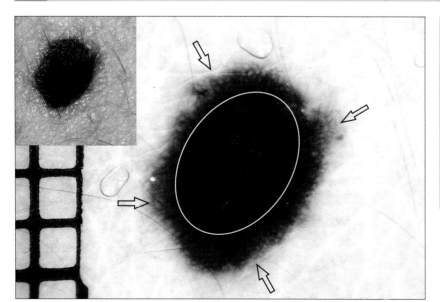

FIVE GLOBAL PATTERNS FOR MELANOCYTIC NEVI	
Reticular pattern	☐
Globular pattern	☐
Homogeneous pattern	☑
Starburst pattern	☐
Non-specific pattern	☐

Figure 91 Nevus

This is a homogeneous type of nevus because most of the lesion looks featureless. Close scrutiny shows hints of dots and globules (arrows) and a delicate pigment network (circle). The white dots represent reflection artefacts from the oil and not milia-like cysts.

FIVE GLOBAL PATTERNS FOR MELANOCYTIC NEVI	
Reticular pattern	☑
Globular pattern	☐
Homogeneous pattern	☑
Starburst pattern	☐
Non-specific pattern	☐

Figure 92 Nevus

This is a homogeneous (circle)–reticular (arrows) type of nevus, commonly called 'black nevus'. A jet-black homogeneous zone ('black lamella') fills most of the lesion, surrounded by a small rim of a typical pigment network. Clinically and dermoscopically this picture simulates an in-situ melanoma and is therefore often excised. Pigmented parakeratosis represents the morphologic substrate of the 'black lamella'. If there are multiple lesions biopsy one to make a dermoscopic clinicopathologic correlation. Tape stripping can be used to try to remove the black lamella.

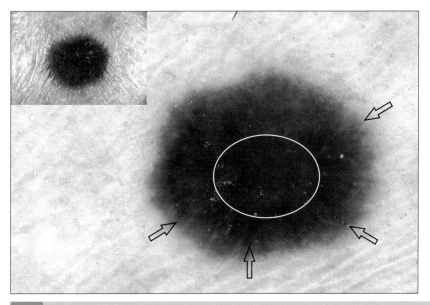

FIVE GLOBAL PATTERNS FOR MELANOCYTIC NEVI

Reticular pattern ☐

Globular pattern ☐

Homogeneous pattern ☑

Starburst pattern ☐

Non-specific pattern ☐

Figure 93 Nevus
This lesion is characterized by diffuse homogeneous pigmentation. There is a subtle rim of radially oriented line segments at the periphery, which represent streaks (arrows), and blue-white structures in the center (circle). The dermoscopic differential diagnosis includes Clark (dysplastic) nevus and Spitz nevus.

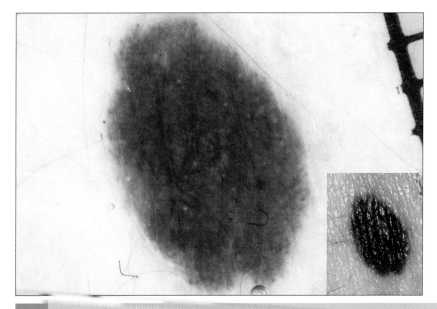

FIVE GLOBAL PATTERNS FOR MELANOCYTIC NEVI

Reticular pattern ☐

Globular pattern ☐

Homogeneous pattern ☑

Starburst pattern ☐

Non-specific pattern ☐

Figure 94 Nevus
Apart from the blue-white structures, this lesion consists of a uniform diffuse brown color characteristic of the homogeneous pattern.

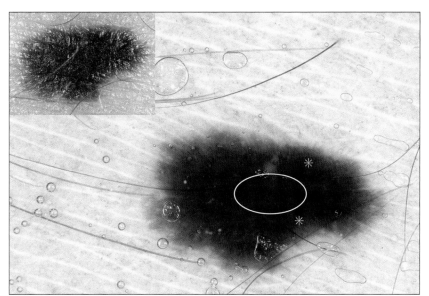

FIVE GLOBAL PATTERNS FOR MELANOCYTIC NEVI

Reticular pattern	☐
Globular pattern	☐
Homogeneous pattern	☑
Starburst pattern	☐
Non-specific pattern	☐

Figure 95 Nevus

A diffuse homogeneous pigmentation is seen throughout this lesion. In the center there are a few dots and globules (circle). At the periphery, a subtle pigment network is seen and there are also blue-white structures (asterisks) throughout the lesion. The latter criterion is the result of macrophages in the papillary dermis. The only striking criterion is the diffuse pigmentation.

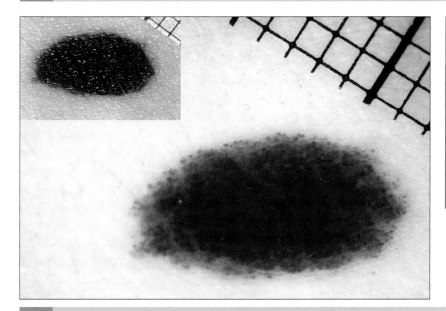

FIVE GLOBAL PATTERNS FOR MELANOCYTIC NEVI

Reticular pattern	☐
Globular pattern	☐
Homogeneous pattern	☑
Starburst pattern	☐
Non-specific pattern	☐

Figure 96 Nevus

A diffuse homogeneous pigmentation fills this lesion. In the center and at the periphery there are a few dots and globules. The only striking criterion is the diffuse pigmentation. One has to look twice to see other features.

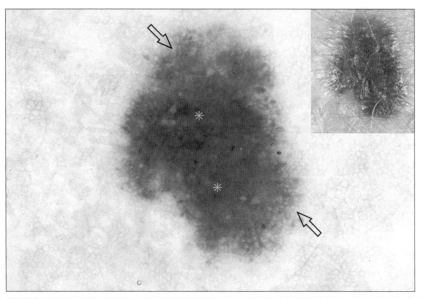

FIVE GLOBAL PATTERNS FOR MELANOCYTIC NEVI

Reticular pattern	✔
Globular pattern	☐
Homogeneous pattern	✔
Starburst pattern	☐
Non-specific pattern	☐

Figure 97 Nevus

This is a reticular (arrows)–homogeneous type of nevus characterized by diffuse brown pigmentation surrounded by a typical pigment network and dots and globules. In addition, there are blue-white structures (asterisks) clearly present in the center. The dermoscopic differential diagnosis includes in-situ melanoma and Clark (dysplastic) nevus.

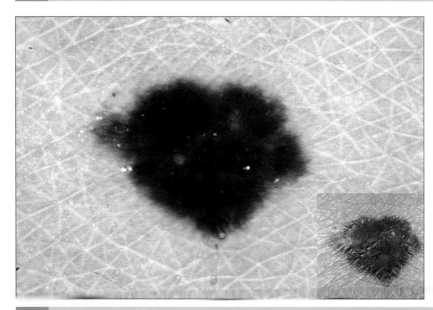

FIVE GLOBAL PATTERNS FOR MELANOCYTIC NEVI

Reticular pattern	✔
Globular pattern	☐
Homogeneous pattern	✔
Starburst pattern	☐
Non-specific pattern	☐

Figure 98 Nevus

This lesion is a variation of the homogeneous –reticular type of nevus reminiscent of a so-called 'black nevus'. Multiple jet-black homogeneous zones are seen at the periphery. Use tape stripping for this black lesion mimicking in-situ melanoma.

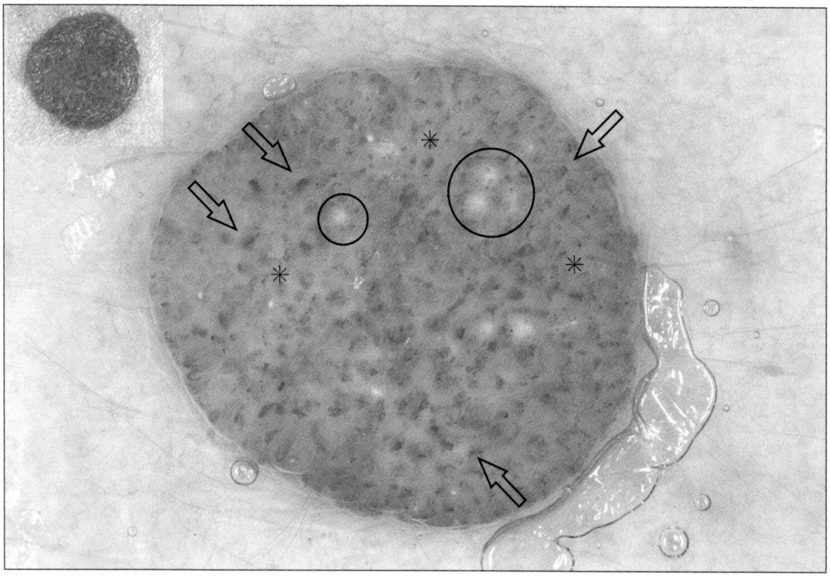

FIVE GLOBAL PATTERNS FOR MELANOCYTIC NEVI

Reticular pattern	☐
Globular pattern	☑
Homogeneous pattern	☐
Starburst pattern	☐
Non-specific pattern	☐

Figure 99 Nevus

This is a dome-shaped melanocytic nevus that reveals a subtle globular pattern with numerous light-brown dots and globules throughout. Multiple blood vessels with dotted (asterisks) and comma-like appearances (arrows) are also seen. There are also a few milia-like cysts (circles), but this is not a seborrheic keratosis. Clinically this lesion could be confused with a basal cell carcinoma, but the vessels in a basal cell carcinoma are thick and branched (arborizing) and there would be no yellow color.

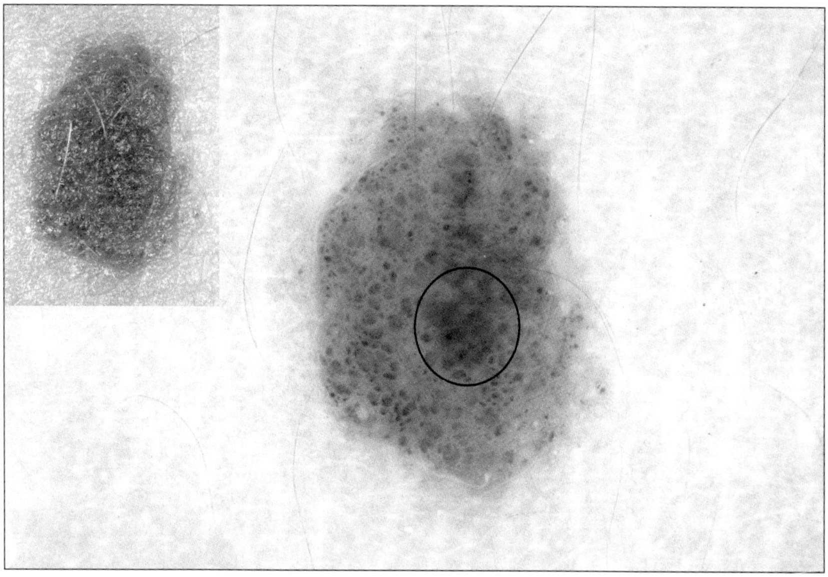

FIVE GLOBAL PATTERNS FOR MELANOCYTIC NEVI

Reticular pattern	☐
Globular pattern	☑
Homogeneous pattern	☐
Starburst pattern	☐
Non-specific pattern	☐

Figure 100 Nevus

This lesion has a globular pattern containing numerous brownish-blue dots and globules, which vary in size and shape, and a central irregular brownish blotch (circle).

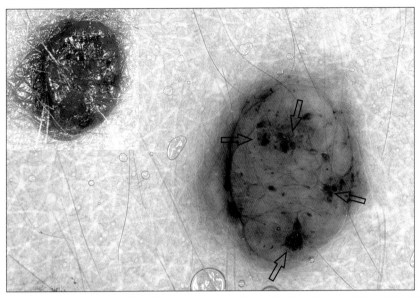

FIVE GLOBAL PATTERNS FOR MELANOCYTIC NEVI	
Reticular pattern	☐
Globular pattern	☑
Homogeneous pattern	☐
Starburst pattern	☐
Non-specific pattern	☐

Figure 101 Nevus

This clinically broad sessile nodule has a papillomatous surface and a few irregularly shaped comedo-like openings (arrows). Sometimes it is not possible to differentiate the comedo-like openings from globules. The thin pigmented lines are not pigment network but pigmentation in the furrows of the lesion. The soft, compressible nature points to it being low risk. Palpate suspicious lesions, but if in doubt cut them out.

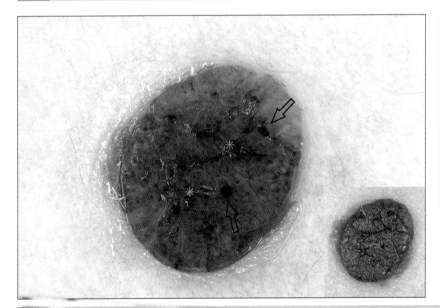

FIVE GLOBAL PATTERNS FOR MELANOCYTIC NEVI	
Reticular pattern	☐
Globular pattern	☑
Homogeneous pattern	☐
Starburst pattern	☐
Non-specific pattern	☐

Figure 102 Nevus

This is another broad, sessile nodule characterized by a papillomatous surface. There are some comedo-like openings (arrows) and a few bluish dots and globules (asterisks). These can be confused with blue-white structures.

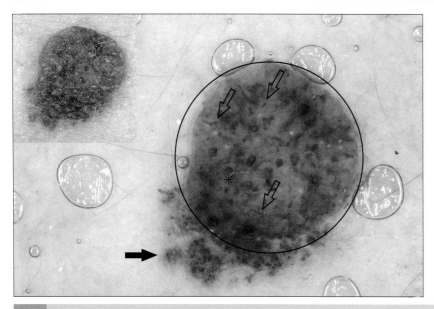

**FIVE GLOBAL
PATTERNS FOR
MELANOCYTIC NEVI**

Reticular pattern	☐
Globular pattern	✔
Homogeneous pattern	☐
Starburst pattern	☐
Non-specific pattern	☐

Figure 103 Nevus

Here is another papillomatous dermal nevus. There are subtle blue-white structures (asterisk) in the lower half of this dome-shaped nodule. This is another lesion to palpate. Compressibility and easy movement from side to side are good clinical signs in favor of a benign nature.

**FIVE GLOBAL
PATTERNS FOR
MELANOCYTIC NEVI**

Reticular pattern	☐
Globular pattern	✔
Homogeneous pattern	☐
Starburst pattern	☐
Non-specific pattern	☐

Figure 104 Nevus

It is common to see a papillomatous nevus (circle) in transition with a flat melanocytic nevus (solid arrow). The flat component can give a worrisome clinical appearance, which in most cases is not high risk when viewed with dermoscopy. The dome-shaped nodule is characterized by numerous comedo-like openings (asterisks). In addition, there are comma-like vessels (open arrows) throughout the lesion. Comma-shaped vessels are not characteristically seen in melanomas. At the lower margin there is a flat brownish area with regular dots and globules.

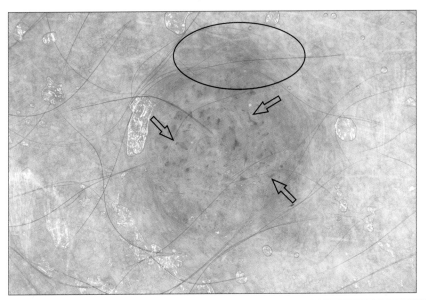

FIVE GLOBAL PATTERNS FOR MELANOCYTIC NEVI

Reticular pattern	☐
Globular pattern	☐
Homogeneous pattern	☐
Starburst pattern	☐
Non-specific pattern	✔

Figure 105 Nevus

This dermal nevus is relatively featureless, but the blood vessels (arrows) might make one consider basal cell carcinoma in the differential diagnosis. The vessels of basal cell carcinoma are linear and branched (arborizing). This slightly elevated dome-shaped nodule has a light-brown to yellowish color and a flat tan macular component (circle).

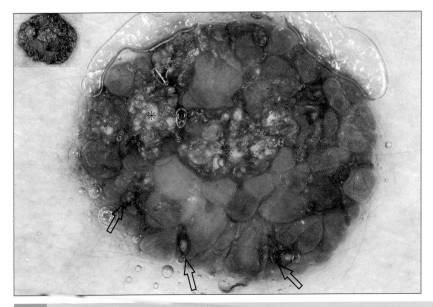

FIVE GLOBAL PATTERNS FOR MELANOCYTIC NEVI

Reticular pattern	☐
Globular pattern	✔
Homogeneous pattern	☐
Starburst pattern	☐
Non-specific pattern	☐

Figure 106 Nevus

In this bizarre dermoscopic picture there are several densely aggregated exophytic papillary structures and ridges, which look like globules. There are also a few irregular crypts and furrows (arrows), which represent a variation of the morphology seen with comedo-like openings. In the center there is an accumulation of yellowish-white keratotic material (asterisks). Palpate this lesion and it will be soft, which will be one criterion in favor of it being a banal nevus.

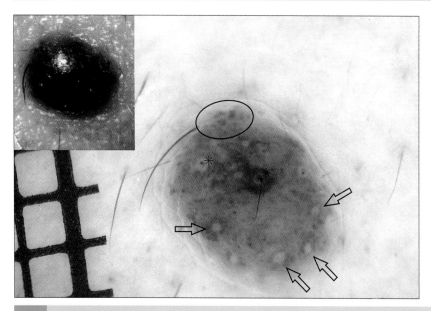

FIVE GLOBAL PATTERNS FOR MELANOCYTIC NEVI

Reticular pattern	☐
Globular pattern	✓
Homogeneous pattern	☐
Starburst pattern	☐
Non-specific pattern	☐

Figure 107 Nevus

This lesion is similar to that in Figure 106 and is composed of densely aggregated exophytic papillary structures intermingled with furrows (asterisks). In addition, there are a few regular brown dots and globules (arrow) and blue-white structures. A small banal reticular-type nevus is seen in the right lower corner.

FIVE GLOBAL PATTERNS FOR MELANOCYTIC NEVI

Reticular pattern	☐
Globular pattern	☐
Homogeneous pattern	☐
Starburst pattern	☐
Non-specific pattern	✓

Figure 108 Nevus

This slightly elevated nevus on the face is characterized by some dark dots and globules (circle). One conspicuous feature is the presence of roundish holes (arrows) representing hair follicles. Closer scrutiny shows hairs (asterisks) in the center of a few follicles. Black pigmentation is seen around one hair follicle, which raises a suspicion of melanoma and justifies excision of this lesion.

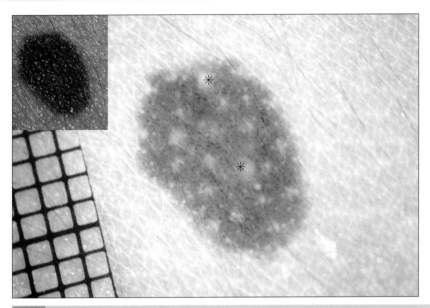

**FIVE GLOBAL
PATTERNS FOR
MELANOCYTIC NEVI**

Reticular pattern ☐

Globular pattern ✔

Homogeneous
pattern ☐

Starburst pattern ☐

Non-specific
pattern ☐

Figure 109 Nevus
Here is a very subtle type of globular pattern in a flat melanocytic nevus with numerous tiny dots and multifocal hypopigmentation (asterisks). This pattern can be seen with congenital or Clark (dysplastic) nevi.

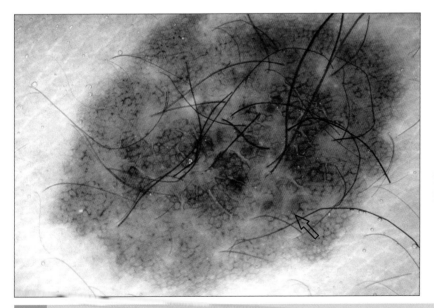

**FIVE GLOBAL
PATTERNS FOR
MELANOCYTIC NEVI**

Reticular pattern ✔

Globular pattern ☐

Homogeneous
pattern ☐

Starburst pattern ☐

Non-specific
pattern ☐

Figure 110 Nevus
This image shows one of the stereotypical patterns seen with congenital nevi. It is a reticular pattern with islands of light, featureless color similar to those seen in Figure 109, but more dramatic. The pigment network in the central portion is more heavily pigmented and the lines are thickened when compared to that at the periphery. There is also a focus of blue-white structures (arrow). Not uncommonly, congenital nevi look worrisome with dermoscopy but histologically they are not. Islands of normal skin + islands of criteria = congenital melanocytic nevus.

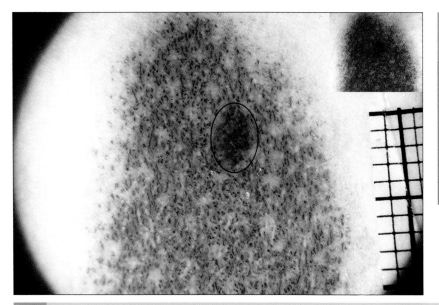

Figure 111 Nevus

The globular pattern seen here is intermingled with roundish white holes and is characterized by numerous tiny bluish dots and globules (circle) situated predominantly in the center of the lesion, and many light brownish globules peripherally. The overall dermoscopic architecture of this lesion is symmetrical and regular and excision is not indicated.

FIVE GLOBAL PATTERNS FOR MELANOCYTIC NEVI

Reticular pattern	☐
Globular pattern	☑
Homogeneous pattern	☐
Starburst pattern	☐
Non-specific pattern	☐

Figure 112 Nevus

This lesion shows another of the many variations of the globular pattern with numerous hypo-pigmented roundish areas. This pattern is very suggestive of a congenital melanocytic nevus. Numerous brownish dots and globules are evenly distributed throughout the lesion. In the upper section there is an oval dark-brown pigmented area. This blotch (circle) could represent high-risk pathology and for this reason the lesion should be excised.

FIVE GLOBAL PATTERNS FOR MELANOCYTIC NEVI

Reticular pattern	☐
Globular pattern	☑
Homogeneous pattern	☐
Starburst pattern	☐
Non-specific pattern	☐

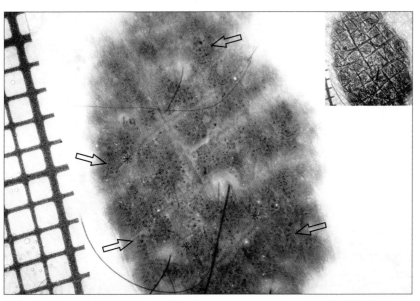

FIVE GLOBAL PATTERNS FOR MELANOCYTIC NEVI

Reticular pattern ☐

Globular pattern ☑

Homogeneous pattern ☐

Starburst pattern ☐

Non-specific pattern ☐

Figure 113 Nevus

This lesion with a globular pattern is a congenital melanocytic nevus simulating melanoma. There is a mixture of dermoscopic features – dots and globules varying in color and shape (arrows), blue-white structures throughout the lesion (asterisks) and a few roundish white areas with hairs in the center. The lower portion of the lesion clearly differs in color and structure from the upper portion and the appearance suggests a superficial melanoma.

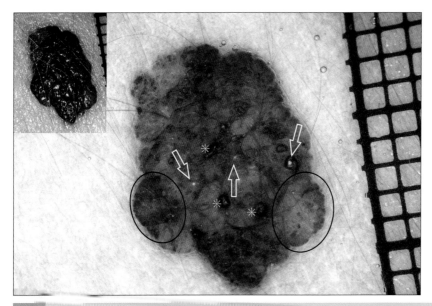

FIVE GLOBAL PATTERNS FOR MELANOCYTIC NEVI

Reticular pattern ☐

Globular pattern ☑

Homogeneous pattern ☐

Starburst pattern ☐

Non-specific pattern ☐

Figure 114 Nevus

This papillomatous nevus is composed of a few exophytic papillary structures (circles) and some comedo-like openings (asterisks). In addition, there are few milia-like cysts (arrows) and blue-white structures. If a worrisome-looking lesion like this is palpated it should be soft and compressible – this sign indicates that it is benign.

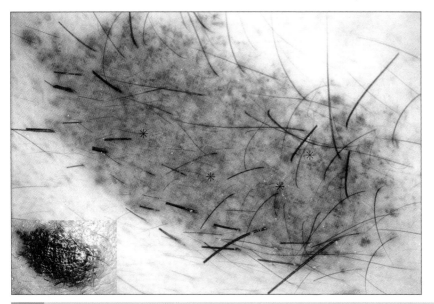

**FIVE GLOBAL
PATTERNS FOR
MELANOCYTIC NEVI**

Reticular pattern	☐
Globular pattern	☑
Homogeneous pattern	☐
Starburst pattern	☐
Non-specific pattern	☐

Figure 115 Nevus

This congenital nevus has a globular pattern, more specifically a cobblestone-like pattern, because the brown globules are angular in shape. Clinically visible but dermoscopically even more pronounced are the skin surface markings, a finding that we consider is never found in melanoma.

**FIVE GLOBAL
PATTERNS FOR
MELANOCYTIC NEVI**

Reticular pattern	☐
Globular pattern	☑
Homogeneous pattern	☐
Starburst pattern	☐
Non-specific pattern	☐

Figure 116 Nevus

This nevus is characterized by the presence of numerous hairs, which is diagnostic of a congenital melanocytic nevus. There are also brownish globules throughout the lesion intermingled with numerous small blue dots (asterisks), which represent collections of melanophages in the papillary dermis and raise the suspicion of a regressing melanoma. Against the dermoscopic diagnosis of melanoma are the presence of multiple hairs and symmetry of color and structure .

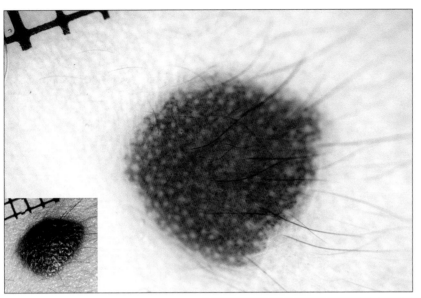

FIVE GLOBAL PATTERNS FOR MELANOCYTIC NEVI	
Reticular pattern	✔
Globular pattern	☐
Homogeneous pattern	☐
Starburst pattern	☐
Non-specific pattern	☐

Figure 117 Nevus

Here is another example of a nevus with dark hairs, which might be best interpreted as a small congenital melanocytic nevus on the face. The dermoscopic hallmark of this lesion is a regular pseudopigment network formed by numerous round areas, which represent follicular openings. This criterion is site-specific. Because of the dermoscopic symmetry of color and structure, a melanoma can be ruled out with certainty. Pigment network is not the same as pseudopigment network.

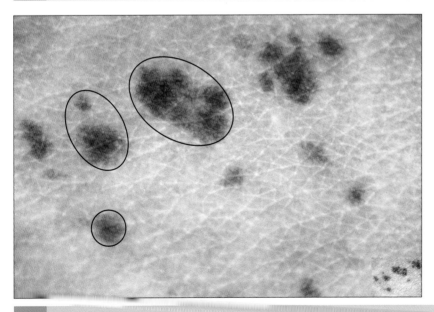

FIVE GLOBAL PATTERNS FOR MELANOCYTIC NEVI	
Reticular pattern	✔
Globular pattern	☐
Homogeneous pattern	☐
Starburst pattern	☐
Non-specific pattern	☐

Figure 118 Nevus

This is a stereotypical example of a nevus spilus, which is characterized by several foci (circles) of a subtle brownish pigment network on a diffuse light-brown background. Each of these spots is reminiscent of a reticular type of nevus. Melanoma can develop in a nevus spilus; therefore dermoscopy is a useful tool for examining these lesions. Look for the same high-risk criteria as for other types of melanocytic nevi.

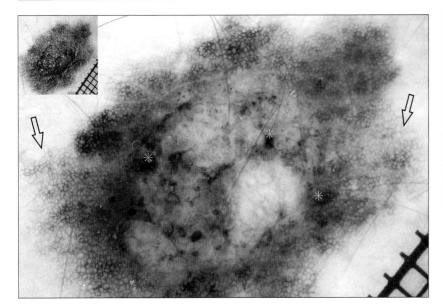

FIVE GLOBAL PATTERNS FOR MELANOCYTIC NEVI

Reticular pattern	✓
Globular pattern	☐
Homogeneous pattern	☐
Starburst pattern	☐
Non-specific pattern	☐

Figure 119 Nevus

This combined congenital nevus has features of a 'normal' congenital melanocytic nevus plus a blue nevus. There are foci of typical pigment network punctuated with a few dark-brown dots and globules (arrows) intermingled with hypopig- mented areas. In the center the roundish blue-white structure (circle) could represent sheets of atypical melanocytes. A biopsy of the heavily pigmented papule is indicated to rule out melanoma arising in a congenital nevus.

FIVE GLOBAL PATTERNS FOR MELANOCYTIC NEVI

Reticular pattern	✓
Globular pattern	☐
Homogeneous pattern	☐
Starburst pattern	☐
Non-specific pattern	☐

Figure 120 Nevus

This congenital nevus has a very worrisome appearance, with a great deal of asymmetry of color and structure. In most areas the pigment network is regular and fades out at the periphery (arrows). There are multiple irregular blotches of pigmen- tation (asterisks) that could be globules or comedo-like openings. Multiple blue-white struc- tures are also seen.

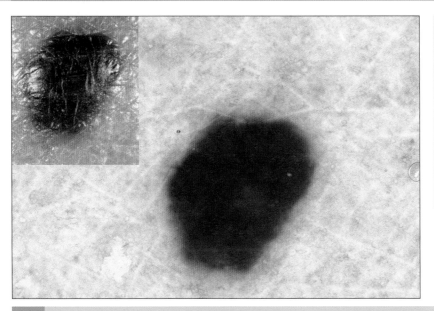

FIVE GLOBAL PATTERNS FOR MELANOCYTIC NEVI	
Reticular pattern	☐
Globular pattern	☐
Homogeneous pattern	✓
Starburst pattern	☐
Non-specific pattern	☐

Figure 121 Nevus

This is a stereotypical example of a blue nevus characterized by diffuse homogeneous pigmentation. There is also a small rim of brownish pigmentation. The differential diagnosis of this blue nevus is a hemangioma, and nodular or cutaneous metastatic melanoma. The history of the lesion is vital to make the correct dermoscopic diagnosis.

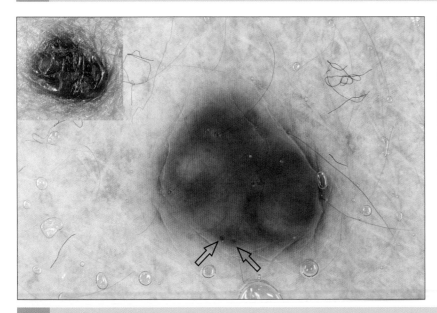

FIVE GLOBAL PATTERNS FOR MELANOCYTIC NEVI	
Reticular pattern	☐
Globular pattern	☐
Homogeneous pattern	✓
Starburst pattern	☐
Non-specific pattern	☐

Figure 122 Nevus

This shows a variation of the morphology seen with a blue nevus. Three different colors are seen: blue, white and brown. There are also two globules (arrows). In this case, the differential diagnosis would include a combined nevus, an atypical dermal nevus and a featureless melanoma. As the lesion may be high risk, it should be excised.

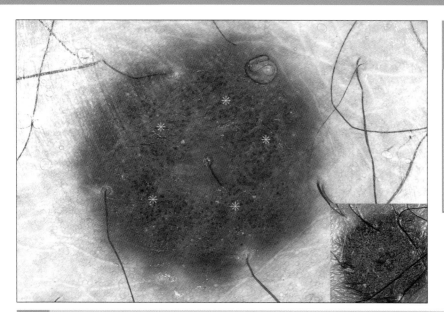

FIVE GLOBAL PATTERNS FOR MELANOCYTIC NEVI	
Reticular pattern	☐
Globular pattern	☑
Homogeneous pattern	☑
Starburst pattern	☐
Non-specific pattern	☐

Figure 123 Nevus

This image shows another variation of the morphology seen with blue nevi and raises important differential diagnostic considerations, such as Clark (dysplastic) nevus with regression and melanoma. The lesion is characterized by a diffuse homogeneous bluish pigmentation throughout, surrounded by a small brownish rim. Numerous tiny brownish dots and globules (asterisks) fill the lesion. These dermoscopic findings are very uncommon in blue nevi and a picture like this warrants a histologic diagnosis.

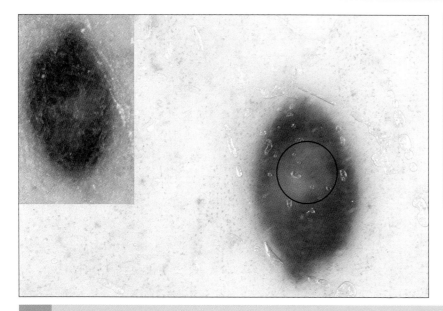

FIVE GLOBAL PATTERNS FOR MELANOCYTIC NEVI	
Reticular pattern	☐
Globular pattern	☐
Homogeneous pattern	☑
Starburst pattern	☐
Non-specific pattern	☐

Figure 124 Nevus

This is a blue nevus with fibrosis (circle) simulating a regressive Clark (dysplastic) nevus or even a regressing melanoma. There is homogeneous blue pigmentation surrounding a whitish area, which corresponds histopathologically to a prominent zone of fibrosis in an otherwise typical blue nevus.

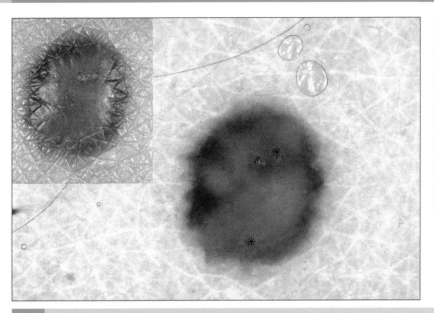

FIVE GLOBAL PATTERNS FOR MELANOCYTIC NEVI

Reticular pattern	☐
Globular pattern	☐
Homogeneous pattern	✔
Starburst pattern	☐
Non-specific pattern	☐

Figure 125 Nevus

This blue nevus is a predominantly firm nodule with a smooth surface. The clinical differential diagnosis includes hypomelanotic melanoma, dermatofibroma or dermal nevus. The nevus has a diffuse light brownish color bordered by small zones of darker pigmentation and blue-white structures (asterisks). No other dermoscopic criteria are seen. Because a hypomelanotic melanoma cannot be ruled out with certainty, a lesion with this dermoscopic picture should be excised.

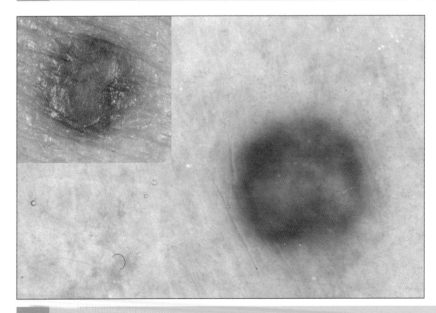

FIVE GLOBAL PATTERNS FOR MELANOCYTIC NEVI

Reticular pattern	☐
Globular pattern	☐
Homogeneous pattern	✔
Starburst pattern	☐
Non-specific pattern	☐

Figure 126 Nevus

This variation of the morphology seen in blue nevi simulates hypomelanotic melanoma and is characterized by a fusion of diffuse bluish and whitish zones. There is a complete lack of individual dermoscopic criteria.

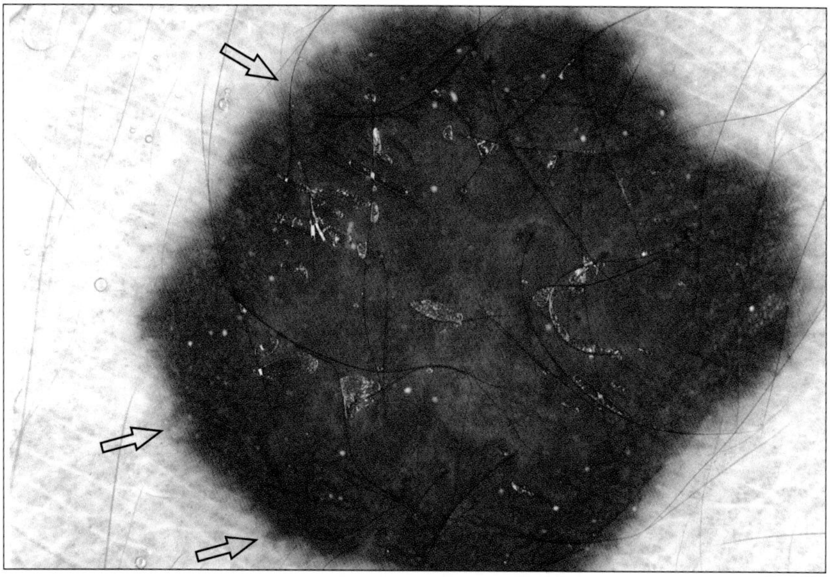

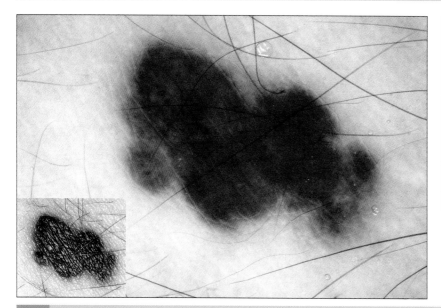

FIVE GLOBAL PATTERNS FOR MELANOCYTIC NEVI

Reticular pattern	☐
Globular pattern	☐
Homogeneous pattern	✔
Starburst pattern	☐
Non-specific pattern	☐

Figure 127 Nevus

This is an example of a blue nevus with diffuse bluish-brown pigmentation. The hint of streaks (arrows) at the periphery of the lesion form a starburst pattern. This could easily be mistaken for a Spitz nevus or nodular melanoma.

FIVE GLOBAL PATTERNS FOR MELANOCYTIC NEVI

Reticular pattern	☐
Globular pattern	☐
Homogeneous pattern	✔
Starburst pattern	☐
Non-specific pattern	☐

Figure 128 Nevus

This lesion is a variation of a blue nevus. Dermoscopically it is characterized by homogeneous blue and gray color surrounded by a faint ring of lighter blue color. There are no hints of local dermoscopic features, particularly melanoma-specific criteria. Nevertheless, because of the lesion's asymmetry of contour and color, excision is justified to rule out a melanoma. The history is also an important factor in this case.

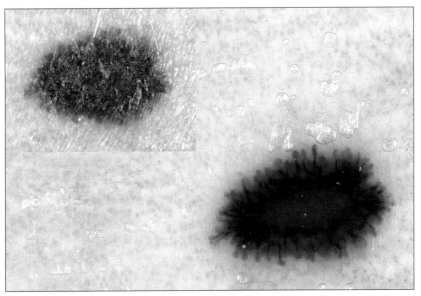

FIVE GLOBAL PATTERNS FOR MELANOCYTIC NEVI

Reticular pattern	☐
Globular pattern	☐
Homogeneous pattern	☐
Starburst pattern	✔
Non-specific pattern	☐

Figure 129 Nevus

This is a stereotypical example of a Spitz nevus with a starburst pattern. There is a symmetrical ring of streaks around the entire lesion and a central blue-white structure. Both these dermoscopic features are commonly found in Spitz nevi. If the streaks are not at all areas of the periphery it could be the dermoscopic picture of a melanoma. A starburst pattern should immediately make one think of Spitz nevus.

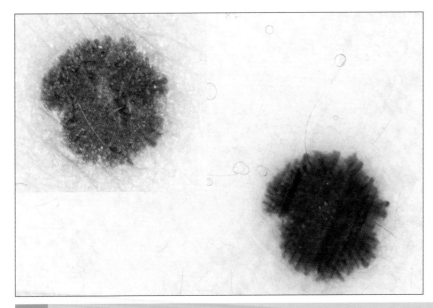

FIVE GLOBAL PATTERNS FOR MELANOCYTIC NEVI

Reticular pattern	☐
Globular pattern	☐
Homogeneous pattern	☐
Starburst pattern	✔
Non-specific pattern	☐

Figure 130 Nevus

This lesion is also spitzoid and similar to that in Figure 129, but the streaks at the periphery are not so dramatic. It also has the starburst pattern. As a rule, excision of a lesion with this dermoscopic appearance is recommended, particularly if the individual is over 14 years of age. The patient can be reassured that in most cases the lesion will not be a melanoma.

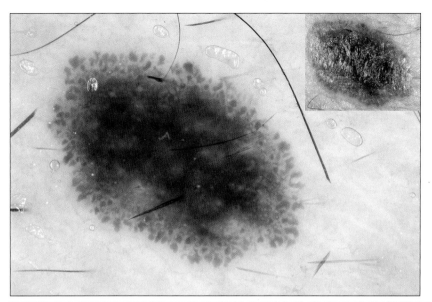

FIVE GLOBAL PATTERNS FOR MELANOCYTIC NEVI	
Reticular pattern	☐
Globular pattern	✔
Homogeneous pattern	☐
Starburst pattern	☐
Non-specific pattern	☐

Figure 131 Nevus

This is predominantly a globular type of Spitz nevus, which dermoscopically raises a suspicion of melanoma. It is a symmetrical lesion characterized by numerous light-brown globules in an annular arrangement at the periphery. A dark irregular blotch fills most of the lesion. The decision about whether to closely follow or excise a lesion that looks like this depends on the clinical setting.

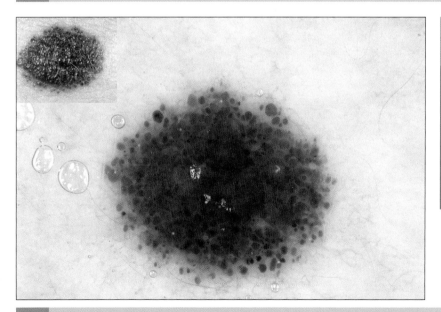

FIVE GLOBAL PATTERNS FOR MELANOCYTIC NEVI	
Reticular pattern	☐
Globular pattern	✔
Homogeneous pattern	☐
Starburst pattern	☐
Non-specific pattern	☐

Figure 132 Nevus

This lesion is similar to that in Figure 71, but the dots and globules, which vary slightly in size and shape, are evenly distributed throughout the lesion. The globules in the center are characterized by a bluish hue because they are situated in the papillary dermis. This globular pattern can be seen in banal, Clark (dysplastic) and Spitz nevi. This was a Spitz nevus. Melanoma can be ruled out with this dermoscopic picture.

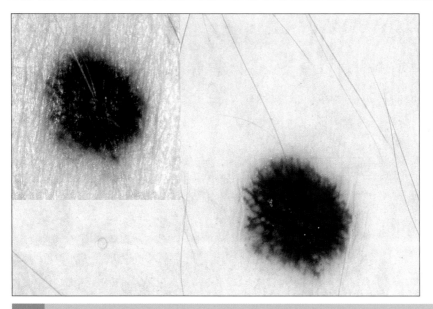

FIVE GLOBAL PATTERNS FOR MELANOCYTIC NEVI

Reticular pattern	☐
Globular pattern	☐
Homogeneous pattern	☐
Starburst pattern	✔
Non-specific pattern	☐

Figure 133 Nevus

This is a very small Spitz nevus. Imagination is needed to see a starburst pattern. There is a thickened and branched pigment network throughout the lesion with an accentuation at the periphery. The differential diagnosis includes Clark (dysplastic) nevus and in-situ melanoma; therefore the lesion should be excised. Small lesions can be high risk.

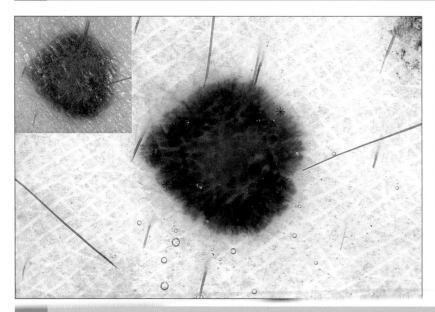

FIVE GLOBAL PATTERNS FOR MELANOCYTIC NEVI

Reticular pattern	☐
Globular pattern	☐
Homogeneous pattern	☐
Starburst pattern	✔
Non-specific pattern	☐

Figure 134 Nevus

This lesion shows another variation of the morphology seen in Spitz nevi. There is dermoscopic symmetry, a blue-white structure in the center, and streaks with a subtle starburst pattern (asterisks) at the periphery. Because a melanoma cannot be ruled out with certainty, this lesion should be excised.

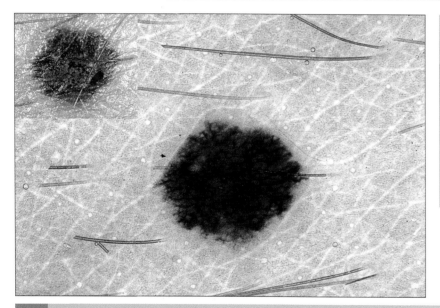

FIVE GLOBAL PATTERNS FOR MELANOCYTIC NEVI

Reticular pattern	☐
Globular pattern	☐
Homogeneous pattern	☐
Starburst pattern	☑
Non-specific pattern	☐

Figure 135 Nevus

The starburst pattern of a Spitz nevus should by now be recognizable. Spitz nevi can have a light or blue-gray dark central area. In this case there is a grayish color with branched streaks at the periphery. The periphery of Spitz nevi can also show dots and globules (circle). The white punctate areas are not milia-like cysts of a seborrheic keratosis but follicular openings. The differential diagnosis of this lesion would be a Clark (dysplastic) nevus or a melanoma; therefore it should be excised.

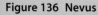

FIVE GLOBAL PATTERNS FOR MELANOCYTIC NEVI

Reticular pattern	☑
Globular pattern	☐
Homogeneous pattern	☐
Starburst pattern	☐
Non-specific pattern	☐

Figure 136 Nevus

This lesion shows another variation of the morphology seen with Spitz nevi. It has a black pigment network with thickened and branched line segments filling the lesion and blue-white structures in the background. There are several highly suggestive spitzoid patterns.

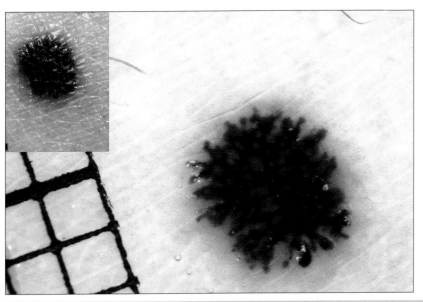

FIVE GLOBAL PATTERNS FOR MELANOCYTIC NEVI

Reticular pattern	☐
Globular pattern	☐
Homogeneous pattern	☐
Starburst pattern	✔
Non-specific pattern	☐

Figure 137 Nevus

Its impossible to see too many variations of Spitz nevi, so here is another classic one! The most remarkable aspect of this lesion is a black pigment network forming streaks that create a starburst pattern. There is also a corona of light pink color surrounding the lesion. The corona is a highly specific sign for Spitz nevi.

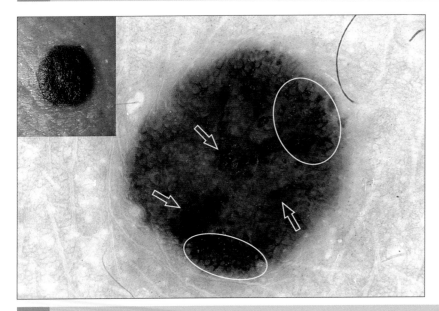

FIVE GLOBAL PATTERNS FOR MELANOCYTIC NEVI

Reticular pattern	☐
Globular pattern	☐
Homogeneous pattern	☐
Starburst pattern	✔
Non-specific pattern	☐

Figure 138 Nevus

This Spitz nevus is not as easy to diagnose as that in Figure 137. It is characterized by several foci of a brown-black pigment network (circles) intermingled with irregular black dots and globules (arrows). There is also diffuse blue-white color – a good example of a blue-white structure. Because of the overall asymmetry of color and structure, melanoma should be ruled out.

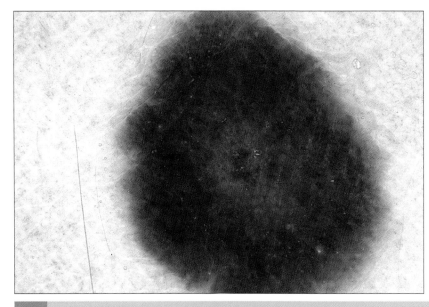

**FIVE GLOBAL
PATTERNS FOR
MELANOCYTIC NEVI**

Reticular pattern	☐
Globular pattern	☐
Homogeneous pattern	☑
Starburst pattern	☐
Non-specific pattern	☐

Figure 139 Nevus

Spitz nevi have many faces! This one is harder to diagnose because the dermoscopic features are not distinctive. It has a central diffuse blue-white structure (circle), streaks (asterisks) and dots and globules (arrows). The dermoscopic differential diagnosis includes a Clark (dysplastic) nevus, Spitz nevus and in-situ melanoma, so it should be excised.

**FIVE GLOBAL
PATTERNS FOR
MELANOCYTIC NEVI**

Reticular pattern	☐
Globular pattern	☐
Homogeneous pattern	☑
Starburst pattern	☐
Non-specific pattern	☐

Figure 140 Nevus

This lesion is similar to that shown in Figure 139, but the criteria are easier to see. This almost structureless lesion has multiple colors – a diffuse blue-white structure and shades of brown. There is no clearcut pigment network. If a lesion cannot be categorized with certainty, then it should be excised to rule out melanoma. The large blue-white structure and symmetry favor a Spitz nevus.

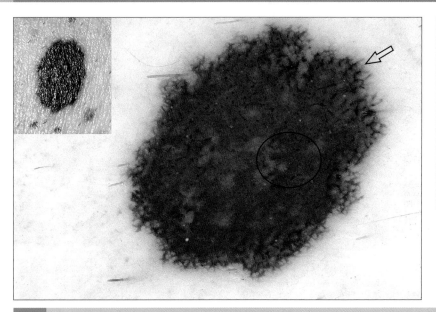

FIVE GLOBAL PATTERNS FOR MELANOCYTIC NEVI

Reticular pattern	✔
Globular pattern	☐
Homogeneous pattern	✔
Starburst pattern	☐
Non-specific pattern	☐

Figure 141 Nevus
This Spitz nevus strongly mimicks a melanoma. Although the lesion is clinically symmetrical, there is some asymmetry of an atypical pigment network at the border of the lesion when looked at carefully with dermoscopy. There are also some streaks (arrow). Asymmetry of criteria favors a melanoma, but as is evident from the diagnosis this is not a melanoma. There is also a homogeneous bluish color filling most of the lesion and some dots and globules (circle). It does not matter whether this lesion is in a child or adult – it should be excised.

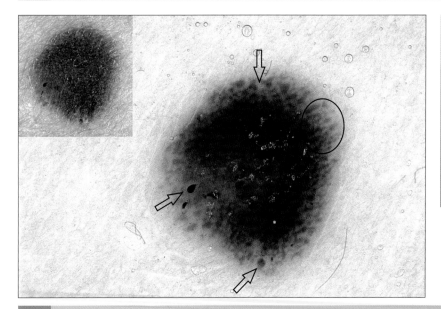

FIVE GLOBAL PATTERNS FOR MELANOCYTIC NEVI

Reticular pattern	☐
Globular pattern	✔
Homogeneous pattern	☐
Starburst pattern	☐
Non-specific pattern	☐

Figure 142 Nevus
This lesion can be categorized as a globular type of Spitz nevus. Because of the asymmetry and multiple colors, it is another lesion that simulates a melanoma. Remember that dermoscopy is not 100% diagnostic for any single lesion. There are numerous asymmetrically located dots and globules (arrows), irregular brown streaks (circle) and blue-white structures.

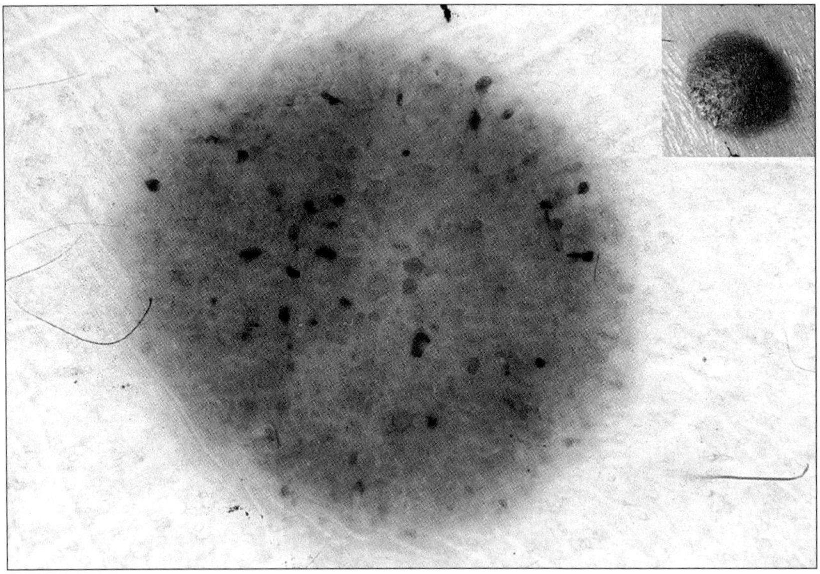

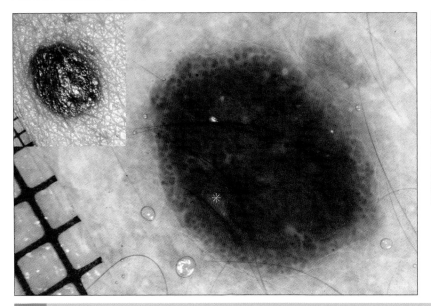

FIVE GLOBAL PATTERNS FOR MELANOCYTIC NEVI

Reticular pattern	☐
Globular pattern	✔
Homogeneous pattern	☐
Starburst pattern	☐
Non-specific pattern	☐

Figure 143 Nevus
This Spitz nevus is characterized by a globular pattern and again mimicks melanoma. There is a central blue-white structure and several irregular brown and black dots and globules, unevenly distributed throughout the lesion, creating structural asymmetry. No pigment network can be identified.

FIVE GLOBAL PATTERNS FOR MELANOCYTIC NEVI

Reticular pattern	☐
Globular pattern	✔
Homogeneous pattern	✔
Starburst pattern	☐
Non-specific pattern	☐

Figure 144 Nevus
On initial impression this lesion should appear high risk because it is so dark. Remember that black color is not always an ominous sign. This is another variation of a homogeneous and globular Spitz nevus. Dermoscopically it is a symmetrical lesion characterized by a large homogeneous central zone of dark pigmentation surrounded by a thin rim of brown dots and globules. A subtle blue-white structure can also be seen (asterisk). Melanoma cannot be ruled out with certainty; therefore this lesion should be excised.

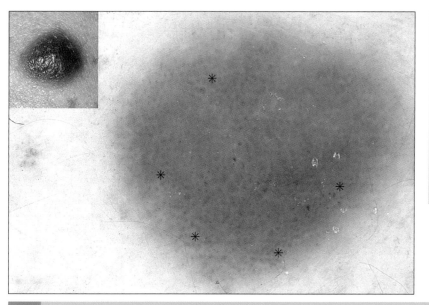

FIVE GLOBAL PATTERNS FOR MELANOCYTIC NEVI

Reticular pattern	☐
Globular pattern	☐
Homogeneous pattern	☐
Starburst pattern	☐
Non-specific pattern	✓

Figure 145 Nevus

A very good dermoscopist might not recognize this as a Spitz nevus without the help of the clinical history. This pink homogeneous type of Spitz nevus is reminiscent of a featureless melanoma with no melanoma-specific criteria. There is light-brown and pinkish pigmentation throughout. There are also a few brown dots and globules (asterisks), but one has to look hard to find them. Relatively featureless pinkish lesions should be excised because occasionally they are melanomas. Pink color beware!

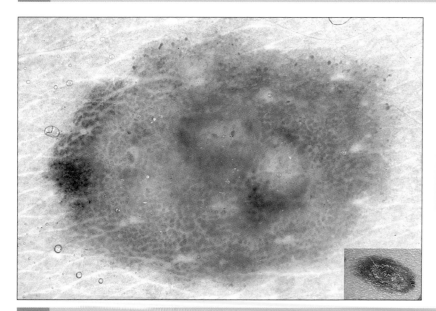

FIVE GLOBAL PATTERNS FOR MELANOCYTIC NEVI

Reticular pattern	☐
Globular pattern	✓
Homogeneous pattern	✓
Starburst pattern	☐
Non-specific pattern	☐

Figure 146 Nevus

This lesion has a totally asymmetrical pattern, yet is another Spitz nevus. There is a large homogeneous central zone, a blue-white structure and asymmetrically located dots and globules. This is a very worrisome pattern and it is surprising that this was not a melanoma.

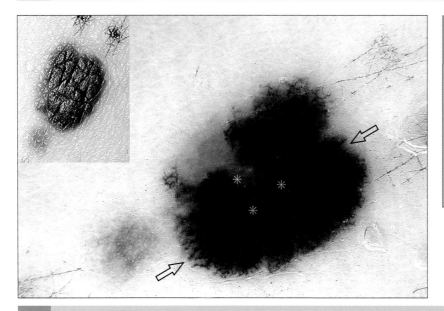

FIVE GLOBAL PATTERNS FOR MELANOCYTIC NEVI

Reticular pattern	☐
Globular pattern	☑
Homogeneous pattern	☑
Starburst pattern	☐
Non-specific pattern	☐

Figure 147 Nevus

This looks worrisome, but is another Spitz nevus simulating melanoma; 20% of Spitz nevi can mimic melanoma clinically and dermoscopically. The most remarkable aspect of this lesion is the dermoscopic asymmetry of color and structure, the presence of central blue-white structures (circle) and unevenly distributed dots and globules (asterisks). The presence of blue-white structures and dermoscopic asymmetry created by the dots and globules points to a high-risk lesion. This lesion needs to be excised.

FIVE GLOBAL PATTERNS FOR MELANOCYTIC NEVI

Reticular pattern	☑
Globular pattern	☐
Homogeneous pattern	☐
Starburst pattern	☐
Non-specific pattern	☐

Figure 148 Nevus

Again this is not a melanoma – it is a Spitz nevus with a superficial black network. This asymmetrical lesion is characterized by a jet-black pigment network with blue-white structures (asterisks) in the background and irregular streaks (arrows) at the periphery. The differential diagnosis includes a Spitz or Clark (dysplastic) nevus and melanoma. If this was a melanoma, it would be in situ or 'early invasive' because the black color indicates that the melanin is high up in the epidermis. Tape strip a lesion like this to see whether this type of black lamella can be removed. If it can, one might see more local dermoscopic criteria.

FIVE PATTERNS FOR ACRAL MELANOCYTIC LESIONS

The parallel pattern is found exclusively in melanocytic lesions on glabrous skin of palms and soles because of the presence of particular anatomic structures inherent to these locations. The pigmentation may follow the furrows as well as the ridges of glabrous skin, but rarely may also be arranged at a right angle to these pre-existing structures:

- the parallel furrow, lattice-like and fibrillar patterns are commonly found in acral benign nevi;
- the parallel ridge and non-specific patterns are suggestive of melanomas on acral sites.

GENERAL DERMOSCOPIC PRINCIPLES FOR EVALUATING ACRAL LESIONS

- First look at the periphery of the lesion to determine where the ridges and furrows are.
- The pigmentation is located in the ridges when the pigmented lines are thicker than the non-pigmented ones and have white dots running along like a string of pearls. It is not always possible to see the string of pearls.
- The appearance of dermoscopic criteria tends to be out of focus on acral areas, owing to the thickness of the skin.
- Other clinical data such as the patient's age and history of the lesion are often essential.

FIVE PATTERNS FOR ACRAL MELANOCYTIC LESIONS

- Parallel furrow
- Parallel ridge
- Lattice-like
- Fibrillar
- Non-specific

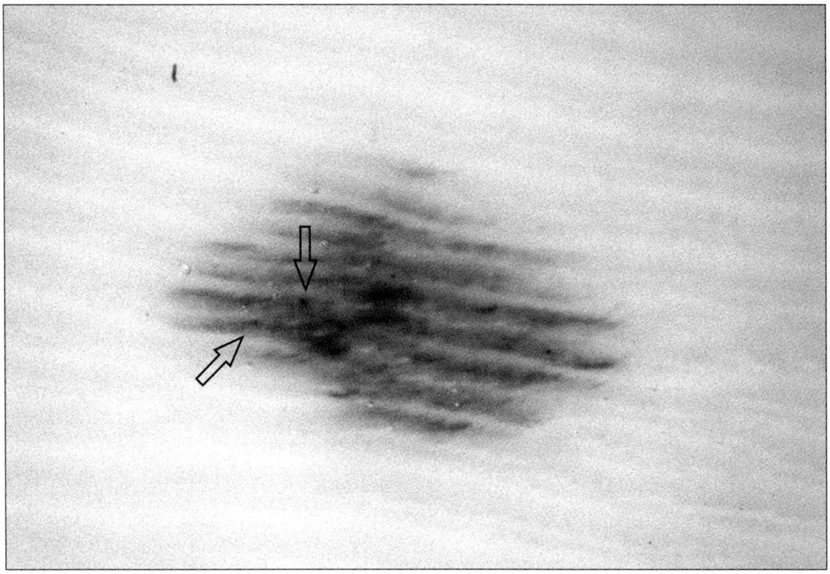

FIVE PATTERNS FOR ACRAL MELANOCYTIC LESIONS

Parallel furrow	✔
Parallel ridge	☐
Lattice-like	☐
Fibrillar	☐
Non-specific	☐

Figure 149 Nevus

This is the parallel furrow pattern of an acral nevus. The dermoscopic hallmark of this lesion is the presence of several parallel pigmented lines in the sulci (or furrows) of glabrous skin. In the center of the lesion, pigmentation is irregular and there are a few tiny dark-brown dots and globules (arrows). Because of the extra pigmentation, the differential diagnosis includes in-situ acral melanoma. It is not always possible to determine whether the pigmentation is in the ridges or the furrows. If in doubt, cut it out!

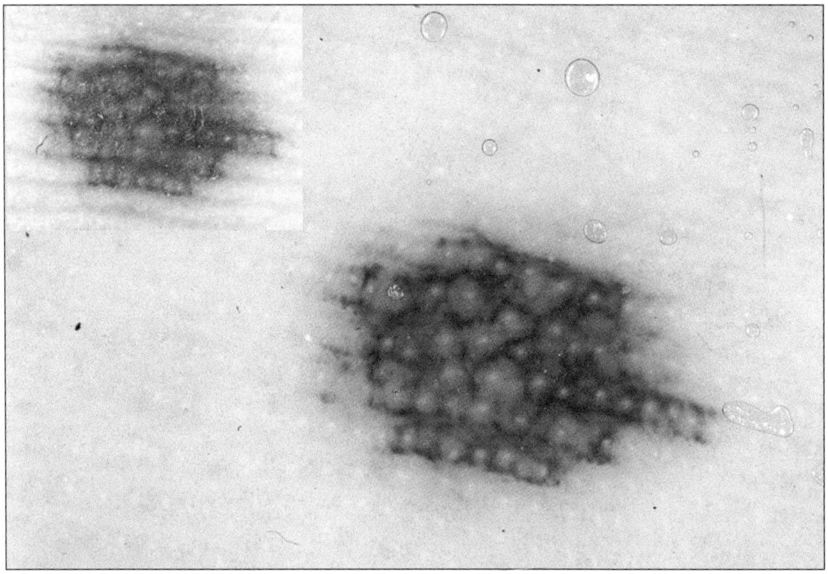

FIVE PATTERNS FOR ACRAL MELANOCYTIC LESIONS

Parallel furrow	☐
Parallel ridge	☐
Lattice-like	✔
Fibrillar	☐
Non-specific	☐

Figure 150 Nevus

This is a stereotypical example of the lattice-like pattern of an acral nevus. It is characterized by a lattice-like structure formed by a rectangular network of brownish lines punctuated by several whitish dots, which look like a string of pearls. The whitish dots represent the openings of the acrosyringia situated in the ridges of the skin. Without specific knowledge of the various dermoscopic patterns of acral nevi this benign lesion could easily be misinterpreted as early melanoma.

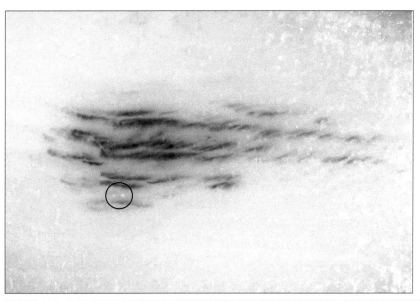

FIVE PATTERNS FOR ACRAL MELANOCYTIC LESIONS

Parallel furrow	✔
Parallel ridge	☐
Lattice-like	☐
Fibrillar	☐
Non-specific	☐

Figure 151 Nevus

This lesion shows a variation of the morphology seen with the parallel furrow pattern, and there are many. There are only a few linear bands of pigmentation following the furrows of the acral skin. The management of acral lesions is strongly influenced by the ability to differentiate the benign parallel furrow pattern from the malignant parallel ridge pattern. Two pearls (circle) identify a ridge.

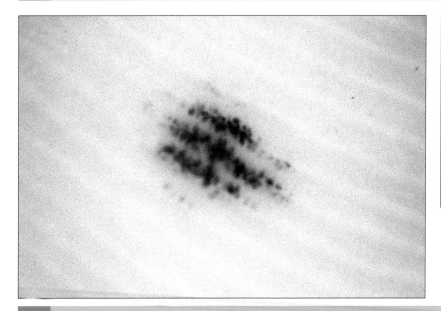

FIVE PATTERNS FOR ACRAL MELANOCYTIC LESIONS

Parallel furrow	✔
Parallel ridge	☐
Lattice-like	☐
Fibrillar	☐
Non-specific	☐

Figure 152 Nevus

Here is another parallel furrow type of acral nevus with a globular component. This very small lesion has only three parallel pigmented lines in the furrows. The pigmented bands are composed of brownish globules arranged in a line. Whatever form the pigment takes in an acral nevus, if it is determined to be in the furrows the lesion is benign. There can be single lines, single rows of dots and globules, and even double rows of lines or double rows of dots and globules. Just ensure the pigmentation is not in the ridges.

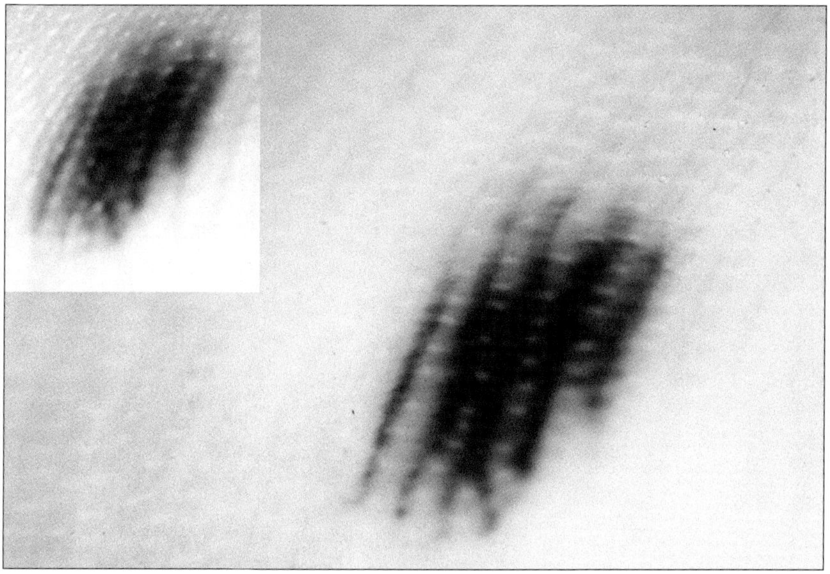

FIVE PATTERNS FOR ACRAL MELANOCYTIC LESIONS

Parallel furrow	☐
Parallel ridge	☐
Lattice-like	✓
Fibrillar	☐
Non-specific	☐

Figure 153 Nevus
This lesion provides another example of the lattice-like pattern. It is composed of a grid of pigmented lines accentuated by numerous whitish dots representing the openings of acrosyringia. The string of pearls is in the ridges. The pigmented lines follow the furrows of the acral skin. Thinner pigmented lines are arranged perpendicular to the thicker lines to form the characteristic lattice-like pattern – like a ladder. There are no criteria to suggest that this might be a high-risk lesion.

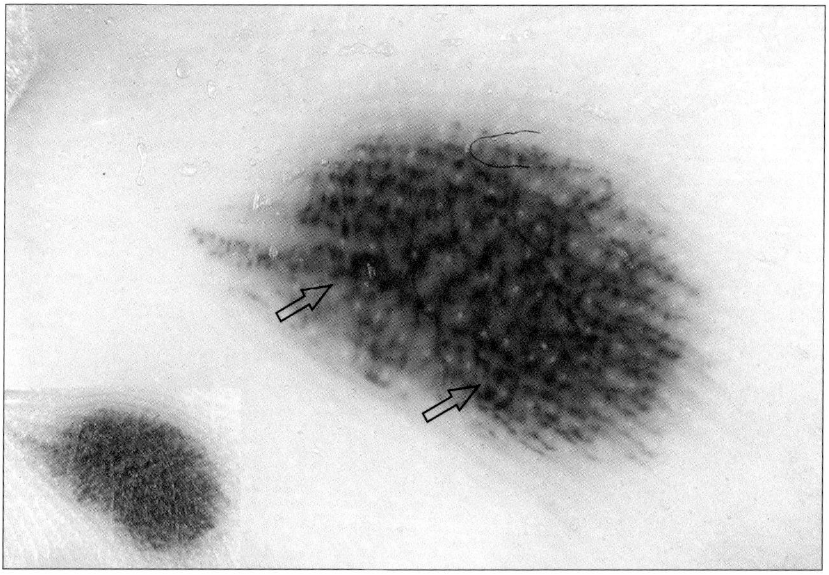

FIVE PATTERNS FOR ACRAL MELANOCYTIC LESIONS

Parallel furrow	☐
Parallel ridge	☐
Lattice-like	✓
Fibrillar	☐
Non-specific	☐

Figure 154 Nevus
Compared to the lesion in Figure 153, this lattice-like acral nevus is harder to define. It is composed of a grid of pigmented lines with multiple whitish dots. The presence of multiple colors (light brown, dark brown, blue-gray and pink), a poorly defined grid and several irregular brownish dots and globules (arrows) makes this a difficult lesion to classify. Pink color beware! Overall these features indicate that this lesion should be excised.

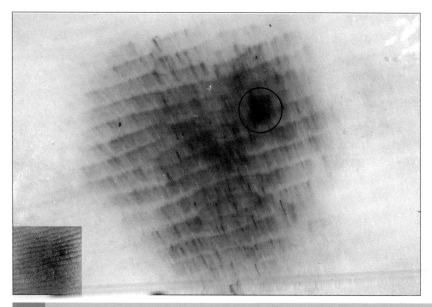

FIVE PATTERNS FOR ACRAL MELANOCYTIC LESIONS	
Parallel furrow	☐
Parallel ridge	☐
Lattice-like	☐
Fibrillar	☑
Non-specific	☐

Figure 155 Nevus

This lesion is out of focus and is a stereotypical example of the fibrillar pattern seen in acral nevi. It is characterized by numerous short and thin brown lines that not only have a parallel arrangement but also run oblique to the ridges and furrows of the acral skin. The parallel furrow, lattice-like and fibrillar patterns are the patterns seen in benign acral melanocytic lesions. Furrow, lattice or fibrillar = benign nevus.

FIVE PATTERNS FOR ACRAL MELANOCYTIC LESIONS	
Parallel furrow	☐
Parallel ridge	☐
Lattice-like	☐
Fibrillar	☑
Non-specific	☐

Figure 156 Nevus

This shows a variation of the fibrillar pattern of acral nevus and it is hard to differentiate this from the parallel ridge pattern. It is composed of numerous, obliquely arranged, smudged, pigmented, thin, short lines. There is also a blotch (circle). Numerous light-brown parallel lines are also found in the furrows of the skin. This lesion is difficult to evaluate; therefore it should be excised. It could easily be mistaken for the parallel ridge pattern, even by an experienced dermoscopist.

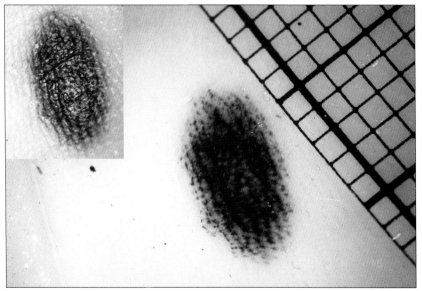

Parallel furrow	☐
Parallel ridge	☐
Lattice-like	☐
Fibrillar	☐
Non-specific	✔

Figure 157 Nevus

This lesion provides an example of the atypical pattern that can be seen in acral nevi and it mimicks melanoma. It is impossible to identify any of the three benign patterns clearly. This lesion is characterized by aggregated globular blue structures (circle) and by a few, light brownish, thin lines following the furrows. Note that there is an interruption of the pigmented lines by the bulk of the lesion. The pinkish color is also worrisome. Excise a lesion with this non-specific pattern.

FIVE PATTERNS FOR ACRAL MELANOCYTIC LESIONS

Parallel furrow	✔
Parallel ridge	☐
Lattice-like	✔
Fibrillar	☐
Non-specific	☐

Figure 158 Nevus

This acral lesion shows many features. It combines parallel furrow and lattice-like patterns. There are parallel lines following the furrows, a grid-like network in the center and numerous brownish dots and globules. The blue-white structure in the center is worrisome. Because this nevus does not fit neatly into any of the three benign categories of acral nevi it should be excised, or the patient should be referred to a more experienced dermoscopist for their opinion.

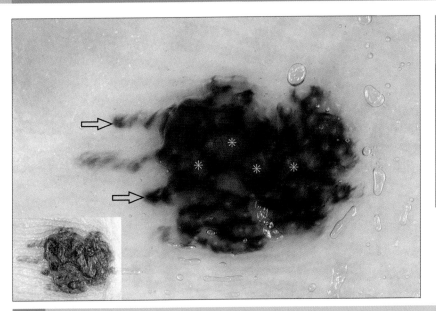

FIVE PATTERNS FOR
ACRAL MELANOCYTIC
LESIONS

Parallel furrow	☐
Parallel ridge	☐
Lattice-like	☐
Fibrillar	☐
Non-specific	✓

Figure 159 Nevus

Here is a clearcut example of an atypical type of acral nevus that dermoscopically simulates melanoma. This asymmetrical lesion is characterized by a pigment pattern mimicking an atypical pigment network and zones with blue-white structures (asterisks). There are also a few dark-brown-to-black dots and globules (arrows) at the periphery. There is no doubt that a dermoscopic picture like this warrants a specific diagnosis. Consider asking for a second pathologic opinion for this type of lesion if the histopathologic diagnosis is not melanoma.

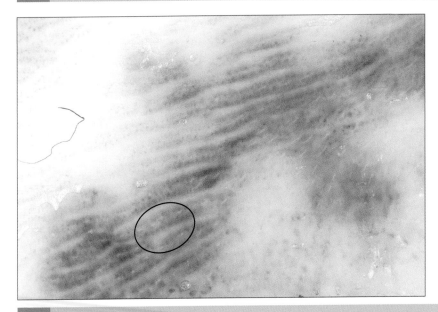

FIVE PATTERNS FOR
ACRAL MELANOCYTIC
LESIONS

Parallel furrow	☐
Parallel ridge	✓
Lattice-like	☐
Fibrillar	☐
Non-specific	☐

Figure 160 Melanoma

This image shows the periphery of an acral melanoma with a parallel ridge pattern. This asymmetrical lesion is composed of several brownish-gray, thickened lines in the ridges of the skin. Note the non-pigmented furrows and string of pearls in a ridge (circle). Remember that the parallel ridge pattern is pathognomonic for acral melanoma. The major pitfall is that the parallel ridge pattern might be misinterpreted as a parallel furrow pattern and the melanoma might be misdiagnosed. Looking at the lesion clinically will often help one decide what to do.

DIAGNOSIS OF MELANOMA USING FIVE MELANOMA-SPECIFIC LOCAL CRITERIA

Melanoma is most often characterized by a multi-component global appearance. The multicomponent pattern is defined as the presence of three or more distinct dermoscopic areas within a given lesion. For example, it might be made up of separate zones of pigment network, clusters of dots and globules, and areas of diffuse hyper- or hypopigmentation. Many combinations of criteria can be seen with this high-risk global pattern. It is highly suggestive of melanoma, but can also be found in basal cell carcinoma. Rarely, it is seen in acquired and congenital nevi and in non-melanocytic lesions, such as seborrheic keratoses or angiokeratomas.

To diagnose melanoma look for the melanoma-specific criteria in a lesion. Melanoma-specific criteria can be seen in benign and malignant lesions, but are more specific for melanomas. Finding one or two is enough to warrant a histopathologic diagnosis.

ATYPICAL PIGMENT NETWORK

A low-risk pigment network can appear as a delicate thin grid or a honeycomb-like pattern of brownish lines over a diffuse light-brown background. Histopathologically, the lines of the pigment network represent elongated and hyperpigmented rete ridges, whereas the lighter areas between the lines are dermal papillae. This criterion represents the dermoscopic hallmark of melanocytic lesions. Alterations are helpful to differentiate between benign and malignant melanocytic proliferations.

An atypical pigment network is characterized by black, brown or gray, thickened and branched line segments, distributed irregularly throughout the lesion. A sharp cut-off of an atypical pigment network at the periphery of a lesion is even more suggestive of melanoma.

IRREGULAR STREAKS

Streaks are dark linear structures of variable thickness found at the periphery of a lesion. The term streaks includes radial streaming and pseudopods, which are variations of the same criterion. Streaks represent discrete, linear, heavily pigmented, junctional nests of atypical melanocytes. Although streaks can be found in benign and malignant melanocytic lesions, they are more specific for melanoma, especially when they are unevenly distributed in a lesion. A symmetrical arrangement of streaks around an entire lesion is most often found in Spitz nevi, but this pattern can also be seen in melanomas.

IRREGULAR DOTS AND GLOBULES

Dots and globules are sharply circumscribed, round-to-oval, variously sized black, brown or gray structures that can be subdivided as regular or irregular based on their size, shape and distribution in a lesion. Irregular dots and globules have different sizes and shapes and are unevenly distributed throughout a lesion. Histopathologically dots and globules may represent aggregations of pigmented melanocytes, melanophages or even clumps of melanin. Dots and globules can be found in benign and malignant melanocytic lesions, and are usually irregular melanomas.

IRREGULAR BLOTCHES

Blotches refer to various shades of diffuse hyperpigmentation that obscure the recognition of other dermoscopic features such as pigment network, dots and globules. Irregular blotches vary in size and shape with irregular borders. A well-demarcated blotch at the periphery is very suggestive of melanoma. Histopathologically blotches represent potentially dissimilar histopathologic structures that share pronounced melanin pigmentation throughout the epidermis and upper dermis. Localized or diffuse regular blotches are suggestive of benign lesions, whereas localized or diffuse irregular blotches favor malignancy.

BLUE-WHITE STRUCTURES

Blue-white structures can appear as white scar-like depigmented areas (bony–milky white color) or bluish structureless areas, or combinations of both colors. Do not confuse white scar-like areas with hypopigmentation commonly seen in benign lesions. Blue-white structures represent an acanthotic epidermis with compact orthokeratosis and pronounced hypergranulosis overlying a large melanin-containing area such as confluent nests of heavily pigmented melanocytes or melanophages in the upper dermis with variable amounts of fibrosis. Whatever color variations are seen, blue-white structures are a high-risk criterion most often found in melanomas. Blue-white structures can also be seen in Spitz and Clark (dysplastic) nevi.

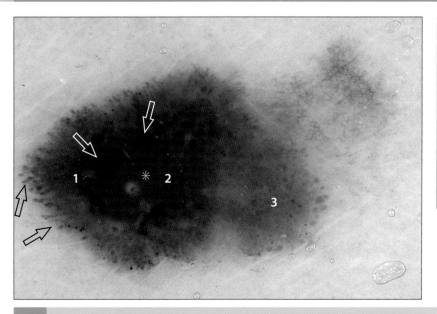

FIVE MELANOMA-SPECIFIC LOCAL CRITERIA

Atypical network	☐
Irregular streaks	☑
Irregular dots/globules	☑
Irregular blotches	☐
Blue-white structures	☑

Figure 161 Melanoma

This melanoma demonstrates significant asymmetry of color and structure, multiple vivid colors and a multicomponent global pattern (1, 2, 3). The melanoma-specific criteria are more than sufficient to make the dermoscopic diagnosis, with asymmetrically located irregular streaks (black arrows), irregular dots and globules (white arrows) and blue structures (asterisk).

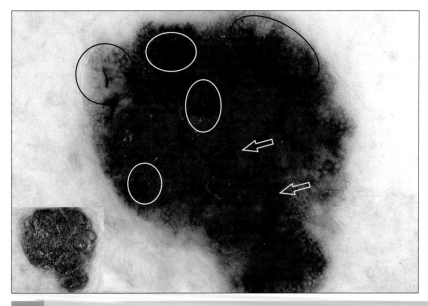

FIVE MELANOMA-SPECIFIC LOCAL CRITERIA

Atypical network	☑
Irregular streaks	☐
Irregular dots/globules	☑
Irregular blotches	☑
Blue-white structures	☑

Figure 162 Melanoma

This lesion also shows significant asymmetry of color and structure and multiple vivid colors. The melanoma-specific criteria found in this lesion include an atypical pigment network (black circles), irregular dots and globules (arrows), irregular blotches (white circles) and blue-white structures.

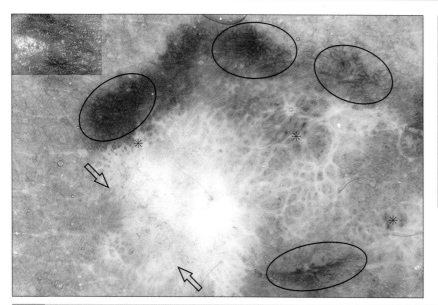

FIVE MELANOMA-SPECIFIC LOCAL CRITERIA

Atypical network	✓
Irregular streaks	☐
Irregular dots/ globules	✓
Irregular blotches	☐
Blue-white structures	✓

Figure 163 Melanoma
The intense bony–milky white color that makes up one component of a blue-white structure is an important clue that this might be a regressive melanoma. There is significant asymmetry of color and structure, though it is not as obvious as in Figures 1 and 2. Melanoma-specific criteria from our algorithm in this lesion include areas with atypical pigment network (circles) and irregular dots and globules (asterisks). On looking closely, some pink color (arrows) can also be seen. The pink color should increase one's index of suspicion that the lesion is high risk. Pink color beware!

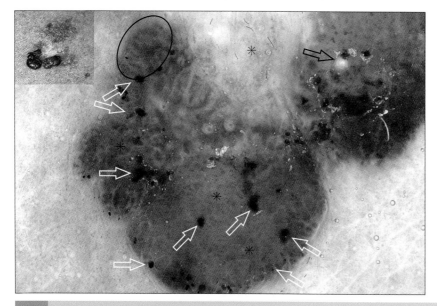

FIVE MELANOMA-SPECIFIC LOCAL CRITERIA

Atypical network	☐
Irregular streaks	✓
Irregular dots/ globules	✓
Irregular blotches	☐
Blue-white structures	✓

Figure 164 Melanoma
This lesion could be diagnosed as a seborrheic keratosis because there are milia-like cysts (black arrow) and irregular dots and globules (white arrows) that could be interpreted as pigmented follicular openings. Once diagnosed as a melanocytic lesion, it will suddenly become very worrisome because there is significant asymmetry of color and structure and a multicomponent global pattern. Melanoma-specific criteria from our algorithm seen here include subtle irregular streaks (circle), irregular dots and globules (white arrows) and blue-white structures (asterisks).

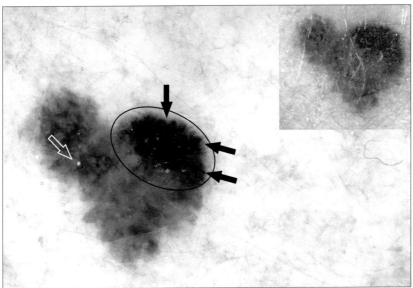

FIVE MELANOMA-SPECIFIC LOCAL CRITERIA	
Atypical network	☐
Irregular streaks	☑
Irregular dots/globules	☐
Irregular blotches	☑
Blue-white structures	☐

Figure 165 Melanoma

The white dots (white arrow) are not milia-like cysts but reflection artifacts from the photography of this lesion under oil immersion. This lesion has only two melanoma-specific criteria. One is obvious – the irregular blotch (circle); and one is hard to find – irregular streaks within the blotch (black arrows).

Always focus attention and look for subtle melanoma-specific criteria in a seemingly benign lesion. The very dark and asymmetrically located irregular blotch is worrisome enough by itself to warrant an excision.

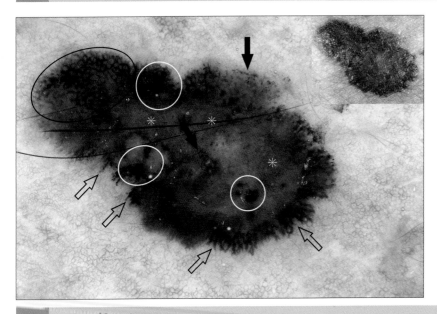

FIVE MELANOMA-SPECIFIC LOCAL CRITERIA	
Atypical network	☑
Irregular streaks	☑
Irregular dots/globules	☑
Irregular blotches	☑
Blue-white structures	☑

Figure 166 Melanoma

This melanoma has all of the melanoma-specific criteria from our algorithm and should be easy to diagnose. There are areas with an atypical pigment network (black circle), irregular streaks asymmetrically located in the lesion (open arrows), irregular dots and globules (solid arrows), irregular blotches (white circles) and blue-white structures (asterisks). Clinically this lesion was in the gray zone of suspicion, but this dermoscopic picture leaves no doubt that this is a melanoma.

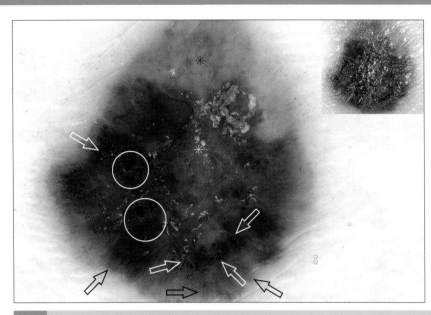

FIVE MELANOMA-SPECIFIC LOCAL CRITERIA

Atypical network	☐
Irregular streaks	☑
Irregular dots/globules	☑
Irregular blotches	☑
Blue-white structures	☑

Figure 167 Melanoma

The obviously present blue-white structures (asterisks) and irregular dots and globules (white arrows) mean that this is a melanoma. If the irregular streaks (black arrows) and irregular blotches (white circles) are missed, the significant asymmetry of color and structure plus the presence of two prominent melanoma-specific criteria should be sufficient clues for the novice dermoscopist to remove a lesion that looks like this.

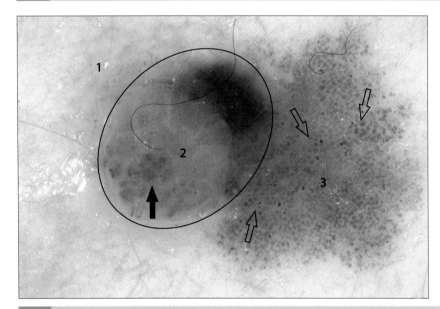

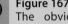

FIVE MELANOMA-SPECIFIC LOCAL CRITERIA

Atypical network	☐
Irregular streaks	☐
Irregular dots/globules	☑
Irregular blotches	☐
Blue-white structures	☑

Figure 168 Melanoma

This melanoma is harder to diagnose than that in Figure 167. The pinkish color (solid arrow), big blue-white structure (circle) and multicomponent global pattern (1, 2, 3) are worrisome criteria. This lesion also has irregular dots and globules (open arrows). This combination of criteria is more than enough to warrant excision.

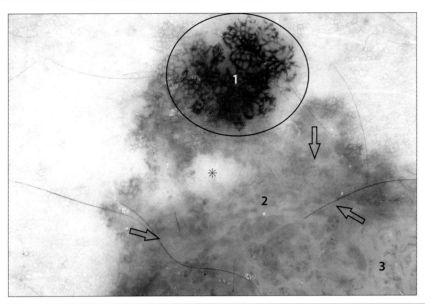

FIVE MELANOMA-SPECIFIC LOCAL CRITERIA	
Atypical network	✔
Irregular streaks	☐
Irregular dots/globules	☐
Irregular blotches	☐
Blue-white structures	✔

Figure 169 Melanoma

The prominent asymmetrically located atypical pigment network (circle) should catch one's eye immediately and make one think that this could be a melanoma. The multicomponent global pattern (1, 2, 3) is also worrisome. Hopefully, the pink color will be seen, which is another important clue (arrows). Pink color – beware! There is also a blue-white structure (asterisk). Interobserver agreement using dermoscopy is not 100% and it is arguable whether a blue-white structure is present because the white color is similar to the white color of the surrounding skin – it should be whiter!

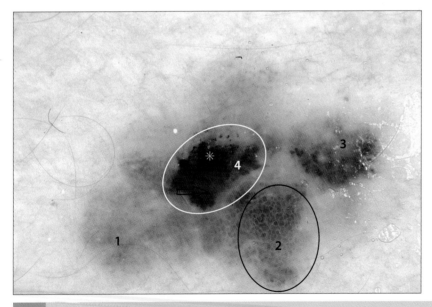

FIVE MELANOMA-SPECIFIC LOCAL CRITERIA	
Atypical network	☐
Irregular streaks	☐
Irregular dots/globules	✔
Irregular blotches	☐
Blue-white structures	✔

Figure 170 Melanoma

This is a melanoma arising in a nevus. The remnants of the globular pattern of the nevus are still evident (black circle). By definition the dark area would not be considered to be an irregular blotch (white circle) because it contains irregular dots and globules (asterisk) and a blue-white structure (arrow). It should be featureless. Two of five melanoma-specific criteria are present plus a multicomponent global pattern (1, 2, 3, 4) and multiple vivid colors. However, no matter how worrisome a dermoscopic picture may look, some of the worst-looking lesions turn out to be benign.

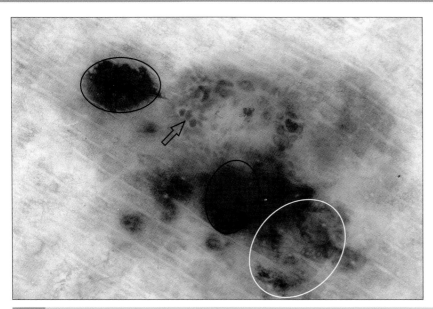

FIVE MELANOMA-SPECIFIC LOCAL CRITERIA	
Atypical network	✔
Irregular streaks	☐
Irregular dots/globules	✔
Irregular blotches	✔
Blue-white structures	✔

Figure 171 Melanoma

This lesion shows only small remnants of an atypical pigment network (white circle). Streaks are nowhere to be found, but there are multiple irregular dots and globules (arrow). Two irregular blotches (black circles) may be considered to be blue-white structures; as they are both high-risk criteria it does not matter if the distinction cannot be made. There is also significant asymmetry of color and structure, a multicomponent global pattern and pink color.

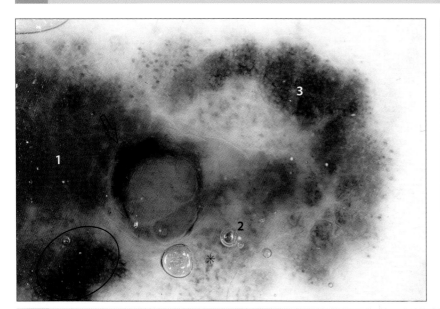

FIVE MELANOMA-SPECIFIC LOCAL CRITERIA	
Atypical network	✔
Irregular streaks	☐
Irregular dots/globules	✔
Irregular blotches	✔
Blue-white structures	✔

Figure 172 Melanoma

It is not necessary to see the entire lesion to know that this is very high risk. It has a multicomponent global pattern (1, 2, 3), asymmetry of color and structure plus multiple vivid colors. The dermoscopic diagnosis is already made. In terms of the list of melanoma-specific criteria there is a dark atypical pigment network (circle) and an irregular blotch (arrow). It is not clear whether there are streaks because the entire lesion cannot be seen; there are irregular dots and globules scattered throughout the lesion; and there is a white blue-white structure. The bluish 'pepper-like' dots (asterisk) are melanophages, which are commonly seen in regressive melanomas.

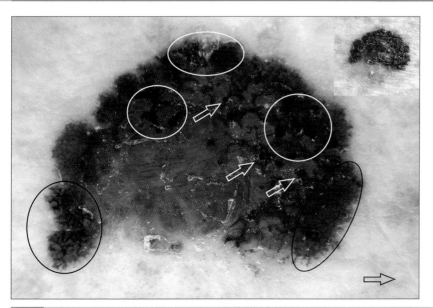

FIVE MELANOMA-SPECIFIC LOCAL CRITERIA	
Atypical network	✔
Irregular streaks	☐
Irregular dots/globules	✔
Irregular blotches	✔
Blue-white structures	✔

Figure 173 Melanoma

It would be very unusual (although not impossible) to see such a vivid blue-white structure and asymmetry of criteria in a benign lesion. There is an atypical pigment network (black circles). Do not confuse the irregular dots and globules (arrows) with the follicular openings of a seborrheic keratosis. There are also several areas with irregular blotches (white circles). This melanoma has four melanoma-specific criteria; some are easy to see and others could be missed. It is not necessary to identify all five criteria to make this dermoscopic diagnosis.

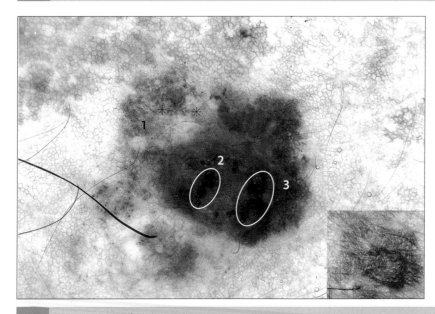

FIVE MELANOMA-SPECIFIC LOCAL CRITERIA	
Atypical network	☐
Irregular streaks	☐
Irregular dots/globules	✔
Irregular blotches	✔
Blue-white structures	✔

Figure 174 Melanoma

This is a small lesion but the blue-white structures and irregular blotches (white circles) make this worrisome. One could argue whether the pigment network is typical or atypical. There are different areas with irregular dots and globules. Some are black and some are bluish and 'pepper-like', representing melanophages (asterisks). The multi-component global pattern (1, 2, 3), blue-white structures and irregular blotches provide more than enough criteria to make the tentative dermoscopic diagnosis of melanoma.

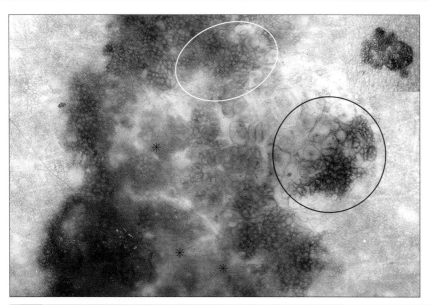

FIVE MELANOMA-SPECIFIC LOCAL CRITERIA	
Atypical network	☑
Irregular streaks	☐
Irregular dots/globules	☐
Irregular blotches	☐
Blue-white structures	☑

Figure 175 Melanoma
The entire lesion cannot be seen, but the white and pink colors should alert the dermoscopist that this could be a melanoma. Now is the time, when the lesion is difficult to diagnose, to go down the list of melanoma-specific criteria to see which are met. There is a good comparision of a typical (white circle) and atypical (black circle) pigment network. No streaks, irregular dots and globules, or blotches are present. The white blue-white structure fills most of the lesion. Remember that interobserver agreement is not 100%, so not everyone will agree with this analysis. This lesion also has pink color (asterisks).

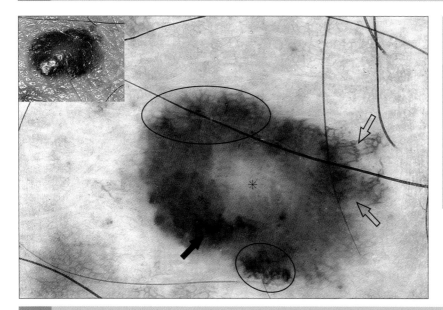

FIVE MELANOMA-SPECIFIC LOCAL CRITERIA	
Atypical network	☑
Irregular streaks	☑
Irregular dots/globules	☑
Irregular blotches	☐
Blue-white structures	☑

Figure 176 Melanoma
Clinically this is a relatively symmetrical lesion, but there is asymmetry of color and structure when viewed with dermoscopy and there is a multicomponent global pattern. The blue-white structure (asterisks) is the most obvious clue that this could be a melanoma. The pigment network is atypical (circles), with a hard-to-see focus of streaks (open arrows). There are also irregular dots and globules (solid arrow). Once again some criteria are easier to see than others.

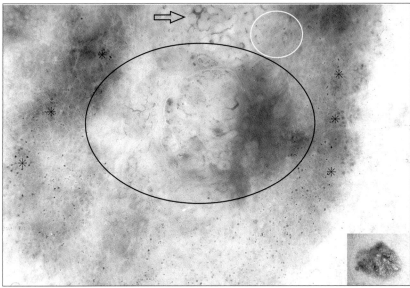

FIVE MELANOMA-SPECIFIC LOCAL CRITERIA

Atypical network	☐
Irregular streaks	☐
Irregular dots/globules	✓
Irregular blotches	☐
Blue-white structures	✓

Figure 177 Melanoma

This light melanoma could be overlooked clinically, but with dermoscopy it is suspicious. Although it has small truncated vessels (arrow) characteristic of a basal cell carcinoma, it is a melanocytic lesion because there are dots and globules (asterisks). There is asymmetry of color and structure plus the multi-component global pattern. From our list of melanoma-specific criteria this lesion has irregular dots and globules (asterisks) and a large blue-white structure (black circle). The vascular pattern most suspicious for melanoma would be dotted and irregular linear vessels (white circle).

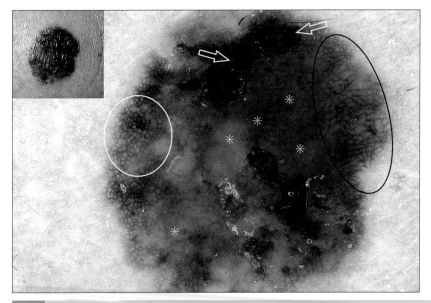

FIVE MELANOMA-SPECIFIC LOCAL CRITERIA

Atypical network	✓
Irregular streaks	☐
Irregular dots/globules	✓
Irregular blotches	✓
Blue-white structures	✓

Figure 178 Melanoma

This image shows many features. A typical pigment network with uniform line segments and holes (white circle) can be compared with an atypical pigment network (black circle) where the line segments are thicker, branched and broken up. No areas with well-defined streaks are seen. Irregular dots and globules with different sizes and shapes are scattered throughout the lesion. There are also several well-developed irregular blotches with irregular sizes and shapes (arrows) located asymmetrically. Blue-white structures fill the lesion (asterisks). Always keep in mind that there are many variations of morphology of the classic dermoscopic criteria.

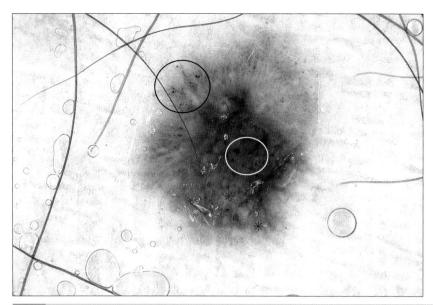

FIVE MELANOMA-SPECIFIC LOCAL CRITERIA	
Atypical network	☐
Irregular streaks	☑
Irregular dots/globules	☑
Irregular blotches	☐
Blue-white structures	☑

Figure 179 Melanoma

This lesion is spitzoid; therefore the dermoscopic differential diagnosis should include a Spitz nevus and melanoma. Do not jump to any rash conclusion that this is a seborrheic keratosis because there seem to be a few milia-like cysts (asterisks). The lesion is spitzoid because there is a starburst appearance of linear brown areas at the borders (black circle). Think of this pattern as being like the spokes that radiate out from the center of a bicycle wheel. Completing the list of melanoma-specific criteria there are irregular dots and globules (white circle) and a blue white structure.

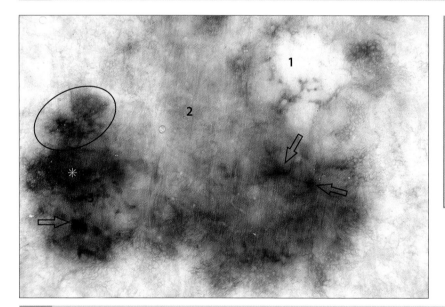

FIVE MELANOMA-SPECIFIC LOCAL CRITERIA	
Atypical network	☑
Irregular streaks	☐
Irregular dots/globules	☑
Irregular blotches	☐
Blue-white structures	☑

Figure 180 Melanoma

The white color should be an immediate clue that this could be a melanoma. There is a difficult-to-find atypical pigment network (circle) and irregular dots and globules (asterisk). The larger ones could be confused with small irregular blotches (arrows). It does not matter if it is difficult to make the differentiation because they are both melanoma-specific criteria. The dermoscopic diagnosis of melanoma in this case will be made because there is significant asymmetry of color and structure, a multicomponent global pattern (1, 2, 3), and a widespread blue-white structure. A lesion with this dermoscopic appearance clearly needs a histopathologic diagnosis.

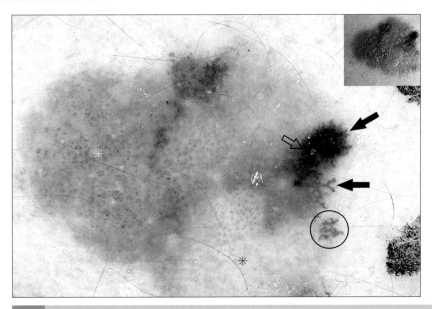

FIVE MELANOMA-SPECIFIC LOCAL CRITERIA	
Atypical network	✔
Irregular streaks	✔
Irregular dots/globules	✔
Irregular blotches	✔
Blue-white structures	☐

Figure 181 Melanoma

This early melanoma is arising in a nevus. The globular pattern made up of uniform dots and globules is the nevus component (white asterisk). There is asymmetry of color and structure with a multicomponent global pattern. Memorizing the list of melanoma-specific criteria will prove useful when looking at a difficult case like this one. An atypical pigment network (circle), irregular streaks (solid arrows) and a blotch (open arrow) make up one small area. There is also a large hypopigmented area (black asterisk) that is not white enough to qualify as a white blue-white structure.

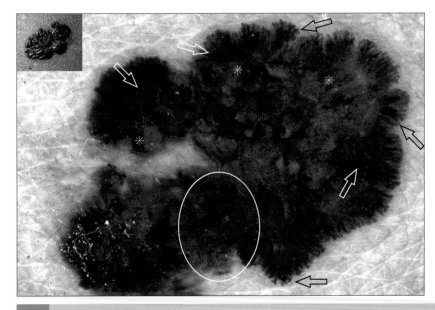

FIVE MELANOMA-SPECIFIC LOCAL CRITERIA	
Atypical network	✔
Irregular streaks	✔
Irregular dots/globules	✔
Irregular blotches	✔
Blue-white structures	✔

Figure 182 Melanoma

This is a very worrisome dermoscopic picture. Some criteria are very easy to see, while others are camouflaged by intense pigmentation and are harder to find. Areas of atypical pigment network (circle) and irregular dots and globules (asterisks) are difficult to see, but will be found if one searches hard enough. There is no comparision between the irregular streaks (black arrows) and irregular blotches (white arrows) seen here and those in Figure 181. There are also well-developed blue-white structures.

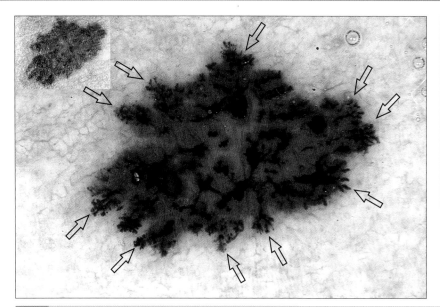

FIVE MELANOMA-SPECIFIC LOCAL CRITERIA

Atypical network	☐
Irregular streaks	☑
Irregular dots/globules	☑
Irregular blotches	☑
Blue-white structures	☑

Figure 183 Melanoma

Spitzoid, starburst, asymmetry of color and structure – this is therefore melanoma. There are streaks (arrows) and areas without streaks. By definition they are irregular streaks, because they are not identified in all areas at the periphery of the lesion. There are also irregular dots and globules and irregular blotches throughout the lesion on a background of blue-white structures.

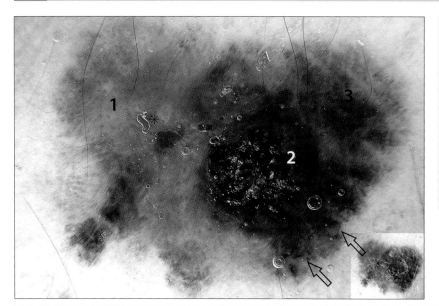

FIVE MELANOMA-SPECIFIC LOCAL CRITERIA

Atypical network	☐
Irregular streaks	☐
Irregular dots/globules	☑
Irregular blotches	☑
Blue-white structures	☑

Figure 184 Melanoma

Pink and black color – beware. Scan the entire lesion. Features include a multicomponent global pattern (1, 2, 3), asymmetry of color and structure, and multiple vivid colors. The pink color shows small red dots and lines (asterisk), which represent the vascular pattern seen in melanoma. Now going down the list of melanoma-specific criteria, there is a barely perceptible pigment network (so it is not considered significant), there are no streaks, there are a few irregular dots and globules (arrows) adjacent to irregular blotches, and blue-white structures are easy to see.

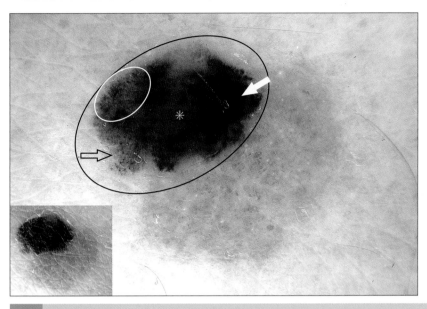

<table>
<tr><td colspan="2">FIVE MELANOMA-SPECIFIC LOCAL CRITERIA</td></tr>
</table>

Atypical network	☐
Irregular streaks	☐
Irregular dots/globules	✓
Irregular blotches	✓
Blue-white structures	✓

Figure 185 Melanoma

Although this is a small lesion, the eccentric area (black circle) indicates the presence of significant activity. The large hypopigmented featureless area is non-specific. The differential diagnosis includes a Clark (dysplastic) nevus and melanoma. There are small foci of pigment network (white circle), irregular dots and globules (open arrow), an irregular blotch (solid arrow) and a blue-white structure (asterisk).

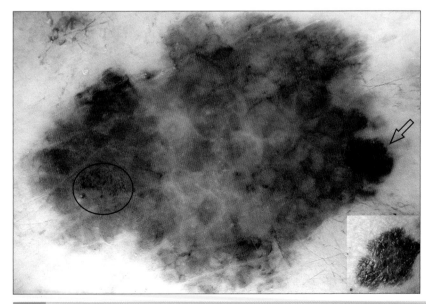

<table>
<tr><td colspan="2">FIVE MELANOMA-SPECIFIC LOCAL CRITERIA</td></tr>
</table>

Atypical network	☐
Irregular streaks	☐
Irregular dots/globules	✓
Irregular blotches	✓
Blue-white structures	✓

Figure 186 Melanoma

This appears to be an easy case – an obvious seborrheic keratosis because there are milia-like cysts. If one is confused, check the lesion against the list of melanoma-specific criteria. Scanning the entire lesion, there is no pigment network and there are no streaks. There are a few dots and globules (circle) with one asymmetrically located irregular blotch (arrow). The blue-white structure is extensive, covering most of the lesion. Significant asymmetry of color and structure and multiple vivid colors are also seen. The dermoscopic diagnosis of melanoma is not difficult if one can recognize the important high-risk criteria.

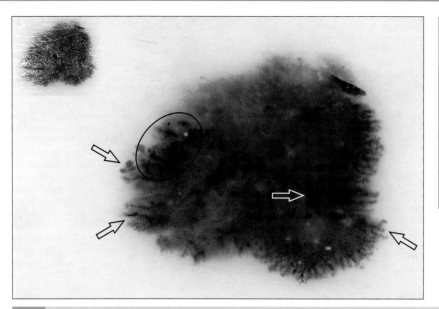

FIVE MELANOMA-SPECIFIC LOCAL CRITERIA

Atypical network	☐
Irregular streaks	☑
Irregular dots/globules	☑
Irregular blotches	☑
Blue-white structures	☑

Figure 187 Melanoma
This spitzoid melanoma is a study of asymmetry, irregular streaks (black arrows) and irregular dots and globules (circle). There are also irregular blotches (white arrow) and blue-white structures.

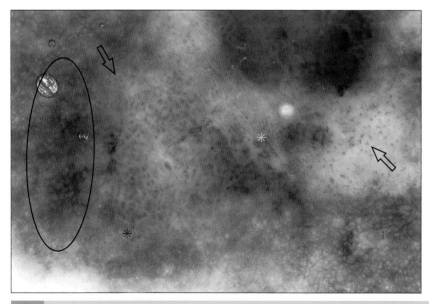

FIVE MELANOMA-SPECIFIC LOCAL CRITERIA

Atypical network	☑
Irregular streaks	☐
Irregular dots/globules	☑
Irregular blotches	☑
Blue-white structures	☑

Figure 188 Melanoma
This is a difficult and subtle case. A lesion that looks like this must not be shaved off because this is an invasive regressive melanoma. There is asymmetry of color and structure with a multicomponent global pattern. There are also foci of atypical pigment network (circle). As the borders of the lesion cannot be seen it is not possible to determine whether there are streaks. There are subtle brown irregular dots and globules (black asterisk) and a blue-white structure (white asterisk). In the area of regression (blue-white structure) there are red dots and irregular linear vessels, the vascular pattern seen in melanoma (arrows). Look for the irregular blotch.

FIVE SITE-SPECIFIC MELANOMA-SPECIFIC CRITERIA

FACE

Annular–granular structures

Annular–granular structures are multiple brown or blue-gray dots (not globules, which are bigger) surrounding the follicular ostia with an annular–granular appearance.

Asymmetrically pigmented follicles

Asymmetrically pigmented follicles are rings of pigmentation distributed asymmetrically around follicular ostia.

Rhomboid structures

Rhomboid structures are thickened areas of pigmentation surrounding the follicular ostia with a rhomboidal appearance (a rhomboid is a parallelogram with unequal angles and sides).

Gray pseudonetwork

Gray pseudonetwork describes gray pigmentation surrounding the follicular ostia formed by the confluence of annular–granular structures. This criterion is rarely seen.

PALMS AND SOLES

Parallel ridge pattern

Pigmentation in the ridges of acral skin must be differentiated from the parallel furrow pattern where pigmentation is in the furrows. The parallel furrow, lattice-like and fibrillar patterns are commonly seen in benign nevi whereas the parallel ridge pattern is diagnostic of melanoma.

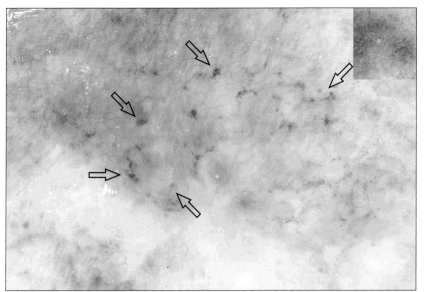

FIVE SITE-SPECIFIC MELANOMA-SPECIFIC CRITERIA

Annular–granular structures	☑
Asymmetrically pigmented follicles	☐
Rhomboidal structures	☐
Gray pseudonetwork	☐
Parallel ridge pattern	☐

Figure 189 Melanoma

Even the most experienced dermoscopist could miss diagnosing a melanoma on the face that looks like this. It is relatively featureless, but there are dermoscopic clues that should convince the dermoscopist to do a biopsy. There are multiple subtle annular–granular structures. In this case they are tiny gray dots (arrows). The color of dots may be gray or brown depending on the depth. The other site-specific criteria for head and neck melanomas are not identifiable. Lentigo maligna could be diagnosed with even fewer criteria, but one should have a high index of suspicion.

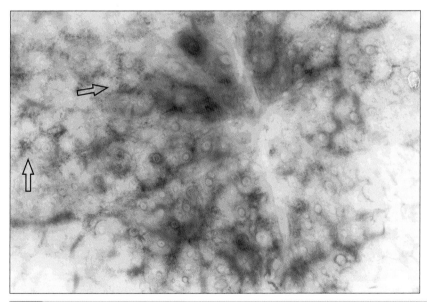

FIVE SITE-SPECIFIC MELANOMA-SPECIFIC CRITERIA

Annular–granular structures	☑
Asymmetrically pigmented follicles	☑
Rhomboidal structures	☐
Gray pseudonetwork	☐
Parallel ridge pattern	☐

Figure 190 Melanoma

Annular–granular structures are present in this lesion and are easier to see than in Figure 189 (arrows). Do not confuse the ostia of the appendages with the milia-like cysts of seborrheic keratosis. Now check the ostia carefully. Some are totally and some are partially ringed by thin layers of pigmentation. The dermoscopic diagnosis of asymmetrically pigmented follicles is made when the rim of pigmentation does not surround the entire ostium. True rhomboid structures are not formed yet. The vessels should not be confused with those seen in basal cell carcinomas. They are a sign of extensive sun damage.

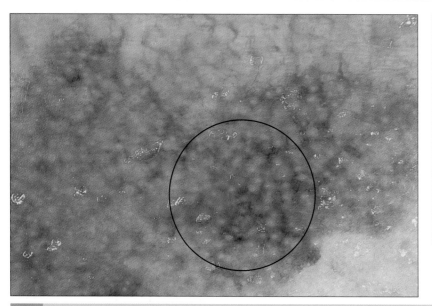

FIVE SITE-SPECIFIC MELANOMA-SPECIFIC CRITERIA	
Annular–granular structures	✓
Asymmetrically pigmented follicles	☐
Rhomboidal structures	✓
Gray pseudonetwork	☐
Parallel ridge pattern	☐

Figure 191 Melanoma

This lesion shows a common variation of the morphology seen with the criteria used to diagnose head and neck melanomas. There are annular–granular structures that are forming rhomboid structures (circle). The gray granules of the annular–granular structures are hard to see, but are there. If true rhomboids, squares or rectangles of pigmentation are seen, a biopsy is needed to rule out melanoma. Annular–granular = rhomboids = gray network.

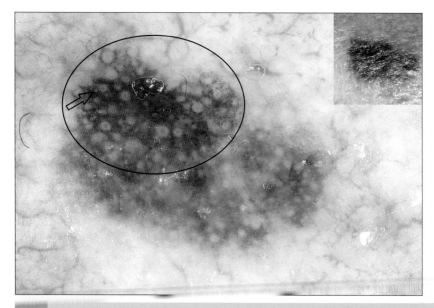

FIVE SITE-SPECIFIC MELANOMA-SPECIFIC CRITERIA	
Annular–granular structures	✓
Asymmetrically pigmented follicles	☐
Rhomboidal structures	✓
Gray pseudonetwork	✓
Parallel ridge pattern	☐

Figure 192 Melanoma

The asymmetry of color and structure seen here should be more than enough for the novice dermoscopist to increase his or her index of suspicion of a high-risk lesion. The annular–granular structures make up rhomboid structures (arrow). Confluence of rhomboid structures makes up the gray pseudonetwork (circle). Biopsy the darker blotch because it could be an area of invasion. Lentigo maligna melanoma – not lentigo maligna. Do not confuse the follicular ostia with milia-like cysts or comedo-like openings.

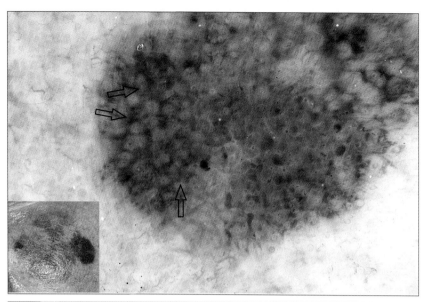

FIVE SITE-SPECIFIC MELANOMA-SPECIFIC CRITERIA	
Annular–granular structures	✓
Asymmetrically pigmented follicles	
Rhomboidal structures	✓
Gray pseudonetwork	
Parallel ridge pattern	

Figure 193 Melanoma

The asymmetry of color and structure plus vivid colors, including an overall pinkish hue, should raise one's index of suspicion that this is a melanoma. Scan the entire lesion for site-specific, melanoma-specific criteria. There are very small annular–granular structures, but no asymmetrically pigmented follicles. There are also multiple subtle rhomboid structures (arrows) and irregular dots and globules. It is possible to see melanoma-specific criteria for trunk and extremity melanomas on the head and neck.

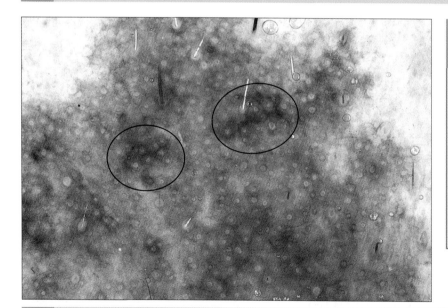

FIVE SITE-SPECIFIC MELANOMA-SPECIFIC CRITERIA	
Annular–granular structures	
Asymmetrically pigmented follicles	✓
Rhomboidal structures	✓
Gray pseudonetwork	
Parallel ridge pattern	

Figure 194 Melanoma

The lesion is from the head or neck because there are multiple white circles, the follicular ostia. If it is thought that these could be the milia-like cysts of a seborrheic keratosis it is a good idea to look at the lesion without dermoscopy. It is flat, brown and not greasy; therefore it does not look like a seborrheic keratosis. Multiple shades of brown color are asymmetrically located in the lesion. The dermoscopic diagnosis of lentigo maligna is made by the presence of multiple asymmetrically pigmented follicles and multiple thick rhomboidal structures (circles).

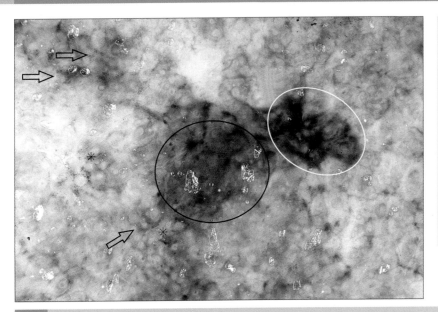

FIVE SITE-SPECIFIC MELANOMA-SPECIFIC CRITERIA

Annular–granular structures	✔
Asymmetrically pigmented follicles	✔
Rhomboidal structures	✔
Gray pseudonetwork	☐
Parallel ridge pattern	☐

Figure 195 Melanoma

If attention is focused only on the bright vivid colors, some of the site-specific, melanoma-specific criteria of this large asymmetrical lesion will be missed. The lighter sections demonstrate multiple asymmetrically pigmented follicles (black arrows), annular–granular and rhomboidal structures (asterisks). Focus attention and remember that it is not possible to see what one does not know. Learn the criteria. The darker section demonstrates asymmetry of color and structure and there is a blue-white structure (black circle) together with more pronounced rhomboidal structures (white circle).

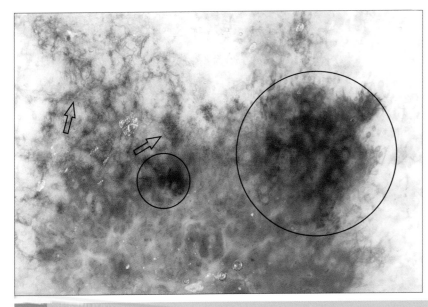

FIVE SITE-SPECIFIC MELANOMA-SPECIFIC CRITERIA

Annular–granular structures	✔
Asymmetrically pigmented follicles	✔
Rhomboidal structures	✔
Gray pseudonetwork	☐
Parallel ridge pattern	☐

Figure 196 Melanoma

Pink color – beware. Asymmetrical lesion – beware. In terms of the list of melanoma-specific, site-specific criteria, there are well-developed annular–granular structures (arrows) and asymmetrically pigmented follicles that blend in with rhomboidal structures (circles). It does not matter whether the criteria are light or dark, if something comes close to meeting the definition of the criteria err on the side of caution and consider them to be present.

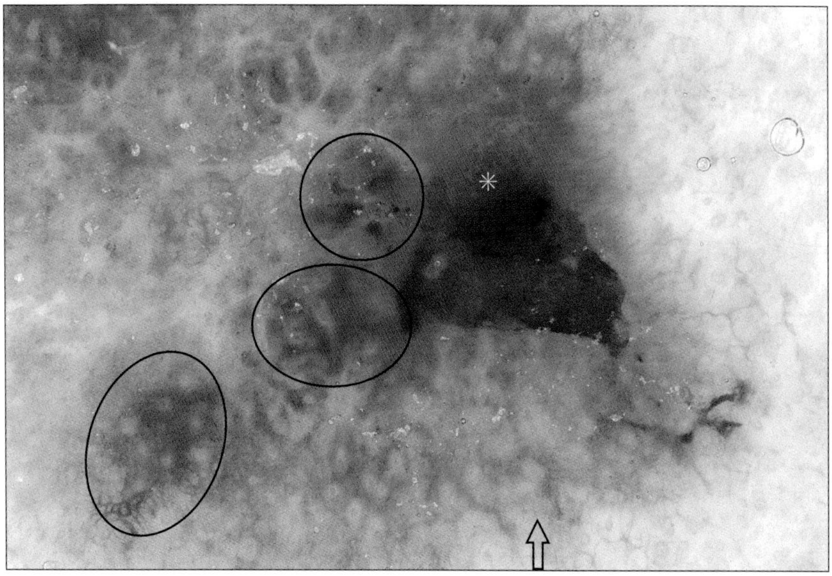

FIVE SITE-SPECIFIC MELANOMA-SPECIFIC CRITERIA	
Annular–granular structures	☐
Asymmetrically pigmented follicles	☐
Rhomboidal structures	✔
Gray pseudonetwork	☐
Parallel ridge pattern	☐

Figure 197 Melanoma

Pink color – beware. Asymmetrical lesion – beware. The blue-white structure (asterisk) is round, but because it is asymmetrically located it is high risk; there is hemorrhage around it. There are some basal cell type vessels (arrow), but focus attention on the network-like structures, which are forming multiple small rhomboids (circles). Remember that to count as a rhomboidal structure, these do not have to be perfect parallelograms with unequal sides and angles. They are rhomboidal structures until proven otherwise. This is not the brain-like pattern of seborrheic keratosis.

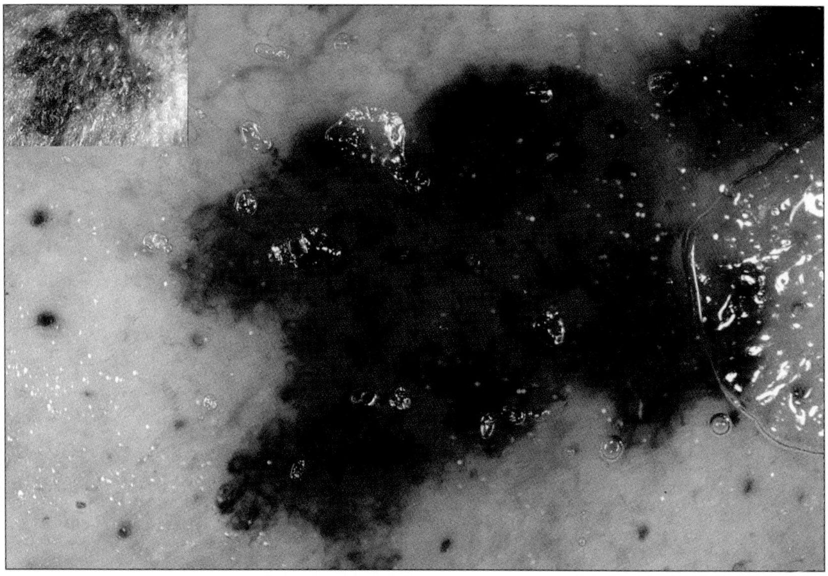

FIVE SITE-SPECIFIC MELANOMA-SPECIFIC CRITERIA	
Annular–granular structures	☐
Asymmetrically pigmented follicles	☐
Rhomboidal structures	☐
Gray pseudonetwork	☐
Parallel ridge pattern	☐

Figure 198 Melanoma

When melanoma becomes invasive, as in this case, the site-specific melanoma-specific criteria are often obscured by intense pigmentation, blue-white structures, and irregular dots and globules.

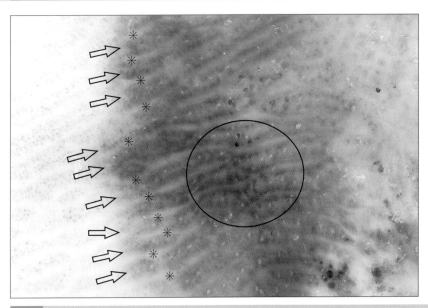

FIVE SITE-SPECIFIC MELANOMA-SPECIFIC CRITERIA

Annular–granular structures	☐
Asymmetrically pigmented follicles	☐
Rhomboidal structures	☐
Gray pseudonetwork	☐
Parallel ridge pattern	✓

Figure 199 Melanoma

Parallel ridge? Parallel furrow? How can one distinguish these two major acral site-specific dermoscopic patterns? This is simple: parallel ridge = melanoma, parallel furrow = benign nevus. The ridges are often thicker (arrows) than furrows (asterisks) and may have little white dots in them. The dots represent sweat ducts and can look like a string of pearls (circle). It is not always possible to differentiate whether the pigment is in the ridges or furrows. Look at the skin without dermoscopy – it might be possible to find both structures. Then try to determine which one has the pigment. If in doubt, cut it out.

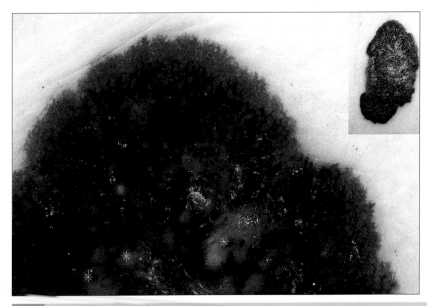

FIVE SITE-SPECIFIC MELANOMA-SPECIFIC CRITERIA

Annular–granular structures	☐
Asymmetrically pigmented follicles	☐
Rhomboidal structures	☐
Gray pseudonetwork	☐
Parallel ridge pattern	☐

Figure 200 Melanoma

This lesion has a very worrisome jet-black color so most likely this is not blood. There are multiple blue-white structures (asterisks). The site-specific melanoma-specific criteria are obliterated by this deeply invasive melanoma.

SIX CRITERIA FOR DIAGNOSING NON-MELANOCYTIC LESIONS

To diagnose non-melanocytic pigmented skin lesions, there should be an absence of criteria for melanocytic lesions (pigment network, globules, streaks, homogeneous and parallel patterns) and the presence of criteria considered specific for basal cell carcinoma, seborrheic keratosis, hemangioma or dermatofibroma.

BLUE-GRAY BLOTCHES

Blue-gray blotches are structureless areas that are round-to-oval and often irregular in shape. The color ranges from brownish-gray to blue-gray. Histopathologically they represent heavily pigmented, solid aggregations of basaloid cells in the papillary dermis of superficial or nodular basal cell carcinoma. Blue-gray blotches are a pathognomonic finding in pigmented basal call carcinoma, especially when associated with arborizing vessels and an absence of criteria seen in melanocytic lesions.

ARBORIZING VESSELS

Arborizing vessels are discrete, thickened and branched red blood vessels that are similar in appearance to the branches of a tree. Histopathologically they represent dilated arterial circulation that feeds the tumor. Arborizing vessels are 99% diagnostic for basal cell carcinoma. Rarely they can be found in intradermal nevi or featureless melanomas.

MILIA-LIKE CYSTS

Milia-like cysts are variously sized, white or yellowish, round structures. Histopathologically, they represent intraepidermal horn globules, also called horn pseudocysts, a common histopathologic finding in acanthotic seborrheic keratosis. Multiple milia-like cysts are predominantly found in seborrheic keratoses, but they can also be seen in papillomatous dermal nevi, and rarely a few milia-like cysts are seen in melanomas.

COMEDO-LIKE OPENINGS

Comedo-like openings refer to brownish-yellow or brown-black, or irregularly shaped, sharply circumscribed structures. Histopathologically, they represent keratin plugs within dilated follicular openings. Due to oxidation of the keratinous material they often have a yellowish-brown or dark-brown-to-black color. Comedo-like openings are found predominantly in seborrheic keratoses, but they can also be seen in papillomatous dermal nevi. At times it is difficult to differentiate dark comedo-like openings from the globules seen in melanocytic lesions.

RED-BLUE LACUNAS

Red lacunas appear as sharply demarcated, round-to-oval structures. The color can vary from red, red-blue, dark-red to black. A whitish color is also often seen in vascular lesions. Histopathologically, red lacunas represent dilated vascular spaces located in the upper dermis. Lacunas with dark-red-to-black color represent vascular spaces that are partially or completely thrombosed. Red lacunas are the stereotypical criterion of hemangiomas and angiokeratomas. Structures similar in appearance can also be seen in subungual and subcorneal hematomas.

CENTRAL WHITE PATCH

The central white patch diagnostic of dermatofibromas, is a well-circumscribed, round-to-oval, sometimes irregularly outlined, milky–bony-white area usually in the center of a firm lesion. There are many variations of the morphology of this criterion.

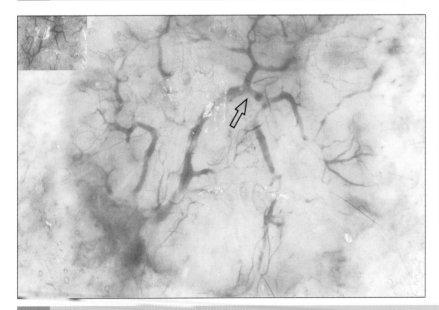

SIX CRITERIA FOR NON-MELANOCYTIC LESIONS	
Blue-gray blotches	✔
Arborizing vessels	☐
Milia-like cysts	☐
Comedo-like openings	☐
Red-blue lacunas	☐
Central white patch	☐

Figure 201 Basal cell carcinoma

Arborizing vessels characteristic of a basal cell carcinoma are hard to see; therefore this could easily be mistaken for a melanoma. The blue-white structures and blue-gray blotches also favor a diagnosis of melanoma, but in this case it turned out to be a basal cell carcinoma. Blue-white structures are found in melanomas, but also in basal cell carcinomas. It is not always possible to differentiate melanoma from basal cell carcinoma with dermoscopy.

SIX CRITERIA FOR NON-MELANOCYTIC LESIONS	
Blue-gray blotches	☐
Arborizing vessels	✔
Milia-like cysts	☐
Comedo-like openings	☐
Red-blue lacunas	☐
Central white patch	☐

Figure 202 Basal cell carcinoma

Do not press down hard on a lesion with vessels like this because they may blanch out. This is a classic dermoscopic picture of a basal cell carcinoma with arborizing vessels (arrow) – like the branches of a big tree! Rarely amelanotic melanoma looks like this. Other criteria are not needed to make the dermoscopic diagnosis of basal cell carinoma.

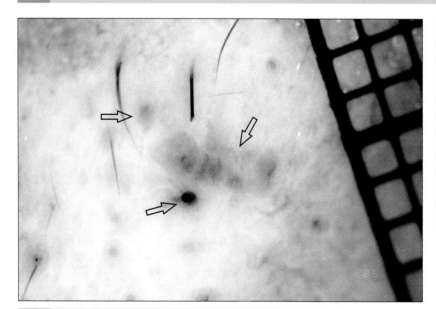

SIX CRITERIA FOR NON-MELANOCYTIC LESIONS

Blue-gray blotches	☑
Arborizing vessels	☑
Milia-like cysts	☐
Comedo-like openings	☐
Red-blue lacunas	☐
Central white patch	☐

Figure 203 Basal cell carcinoma
There is an absence of criteria in this lesion to diagnose a melanocytic lesion; therefore look for criteria to diagnose a non-melanocytic lesion.

Arborizing vessels and a blue-gray blotch (circle) lead to the diagnosis of basal cell carcinoma.

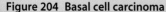

SIX CRITERIA FOR NON-MELANOCYTIC LESIONS

Blue-gray blotches	☑
Arborizing vessels	☑
Milia-like cysts	☐
Comedo-like openings	☐
Red-blue lacunas	☐
Central white patch	☐

Figure 204 Basal cell carcinoma
This is a tiny lesion, but once the dermoscopist has seen a few like this the diagnosis is easy. There are blotches with different shades of blue-gray color (arrows) and some smaller blood vessels. The

differential diagnosis includes a blue nevus and a tattoo. The age of the patient and the history of the lesion are important.

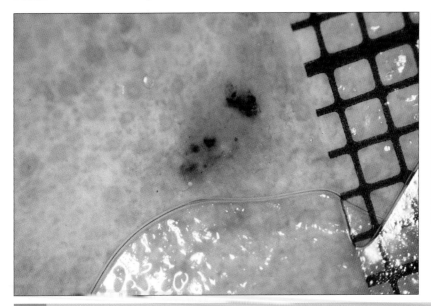

SIX CRITERIA FOR NON-MELANOCYTIC LESIONS

Blue-gray blotches	✔
Arborizing vessels	☐
Milia-like cysts	☐
Comedo-like openings	☐
Red-blue lacunas	☐
Central white patch	☐

Figure 205 Basal cell carcinoma

Pink color – beware. Develop a dermoscopic differential diagnosis because not all cases are clearcut. There is an absence of criteria to diagnose a melanocytic lesion; therefore the next step is to consider which non-melanocytic lesion this is. It does not look like seborrheic keratosis, dermato- fibroma or hemangioma; therefore it would be a basal cell carcinoma. There are multiple globules of pigment (asterisks), also called blue-gray blotches, and there is some ulceration (arrows), which favor a diagnosis of basal cell carcinoma. The lesion lacks arborizing vessels, which is against a basal cell carcinoma. Melanoma could also look like this.

SIX CRITERIA FOR NON-MELANOCYTIC LESIONS

Blue-gray blotches	✔
Arborizing vessels	☐
Milia-like cysts	☐
Comedo-like openings	☐
Red-blue lacunas	☐
Central white patch	☐

Figure 206 Basal cell carcinoma

This is another difficult lesion to diagnose, so the approach would be the same as for that in Figure 205. The clinical appearance will help make the diagnosis in this case because the lesion is a small clear papule. There are no arborizing vessels, just specks of pigment, both brown and gray. There are many variations of the morphology seen with stereotypical blue-gray blotches. The entire picture points to a lesion that should be excised.

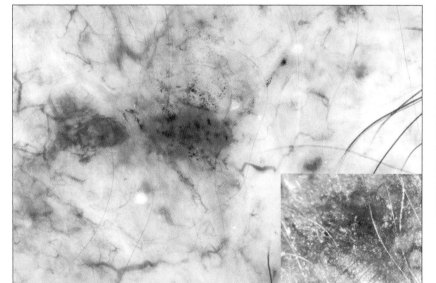

SIX CRITERIA FOR NON-MELANOCYTIC LESIONS	
Blue-gray blotches	✔
Arborizing vessels	✔
Milia-like cysts	☐
Comedo-like openings	☐
Red-blue lacunas	☐
Central white patch	☐

Figure 207 Basal cell carcinoma
This is a stereotypical basal cell carcinoma with arborizing vessels and several blue-gray blotches.

SIX CRITERIA FOR NON-MELANOCYTIC LESIONS	
Blue-gray blotches	✔
Arborizing vessels	✔
Milia-like cysts	☐
Comedo-like openings	☐
Red-blue lacunas	☐
Central white patch	☐

Figure 208 Basal cell carcinoma
Once again this is a clear papule with blotches of gray pigmentation and typical arborizing vessels. The dots and globules could lead to a diagnosis of amelanotic melanoma. There are many variations of pigmentation that can be seen in a basal cell carcinoma; these are generally classified as blue-gray blotches.

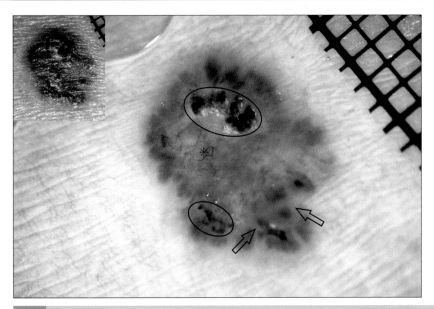

SIX CRITERIA FOR NON-MELANOCYTIC LESIONS	
Blue-gray blotches	✔
Arborizing vessels	✔
Milia-like cysts	☐
Comedo-like openings	☐
Red-blue lacunas	☐
Central white patch	☐

Figure 209 Basal cell carcinoma

This lesion has three criteria diagnostic for a basal cell carcinoma – ulceration (circles), arborizing vessels (asterisk) and blue-gray blotches (arrows). For a novice, the pattern of this lesion might seem similar to the starburst pattern seen in Spitz nevi, but arborizing blood vessels and ulceration are never found in Spitz nevi.

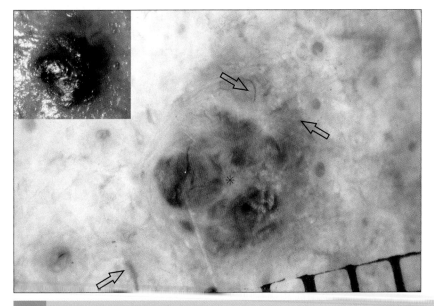

SIX CRITERIA FOR NON-MELANOCYTIC LESIONS	
Blue-gray blotches	✔
Arborizing vessels	☐
Milia-like cysts	☐
Comedo-like openings	☐
Red-blue lacunas	☐
Central white patch	☐

Figure 210 Basal cell carcinoma

In this lesion there are blue-gray blotches, a blue-white structure (asterisk) and sharply outlined blood vessels (arrows). The differential diagnosis includes basal cell carcinoma, atypical blue nevus and a nodular melanoma. The blood vessels (arrows) favor a diagnosis of basal cell carcinoma even though they are not stereotypical branching vessels.

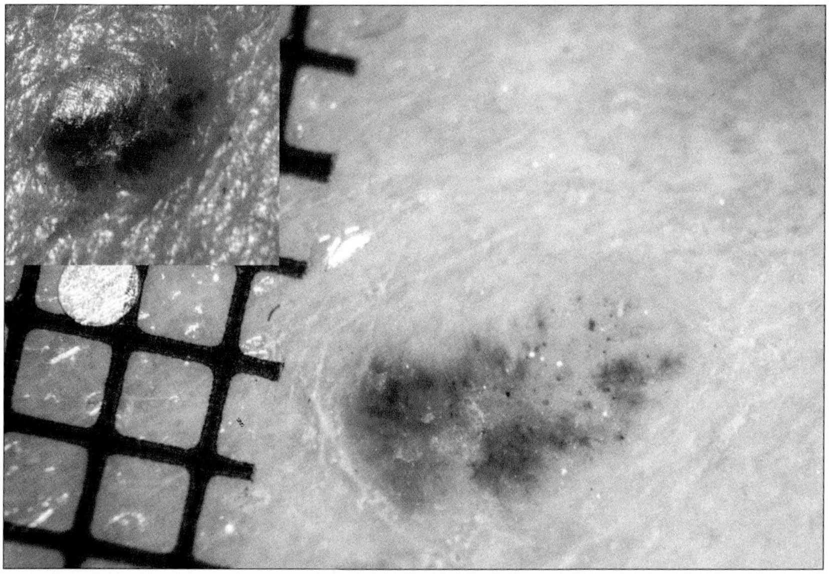

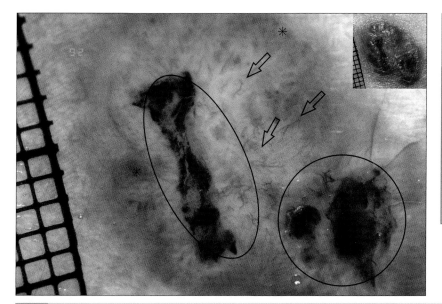

SIX CRITERIA FOR NON-MELANOCYTIC LESIONS	
Blue-gray blotches	✔
Arborizing vessels	☐
Milia-like cysts	☐
Comedo-like openings	☐
Red-blue lacunas	☐
Central white patch	☐

Figure 211 Basal cell carcinoma

This is another small lesion characterized by pigmentation. Multiple pepper-like grayish dots are forming the blue-gray blotches. Criteria to diagnose a melanocytic lesion are lacking. The asymmetry of color and structure and the clinical appearance should be sufficient to warrant a histopathologic diagnosis.

SIX CRITERIA FOR NON-MELANOCYTIC LESIONS	
Blue-gray blotches	✔
Arborizing vessels	✔
Milia-like cysts	☐
Comedo-like openings	☐
Red-blue lacunas	☐
Central white patch	☐

Figure 212 Basal cell carcinoma

Here is another basal cell carcinoma with areas of ulceration (circles), arborizing blood vessels (arrows) and blue-gray blotches (asterisks). This is a clearcut case, but do not forget to develop a dermoscopic differential diagnosis because there will be surprises from time to time.

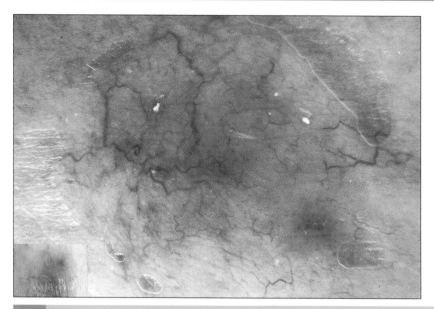

SIX CRITERIA FOR NON-MELANOCYTIC LESIONS

Blue-gray blotches	☐
Arborizing vessels	✔
Milia-like cysts	☐
Comedo-like openings	☐
Red-blue lacunas	☐
Central white patch	☐

Figure 213 Basal cell carcinoma
This shows another variation of the morphology seen with a basal cell carcinoma. Statistically this dermoscopic picture will be a basal cell carcinoma, but amelanotic melanoma can also look like this.

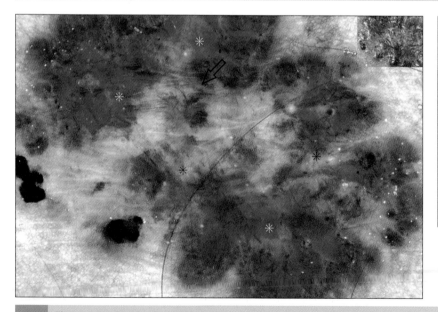

SIX CRITERIA FOR NON-MELANOCYTIC LESIONS

Blue-gray blotches	✔
Arborizing vessels	✔
Milia-like cysts	☐
Comedo-like openings	☐
Red-blue lacunas	☐
Central white patch	☐

Figure 214 Basal cell carcinoma
With this striking appearance, this lesion must be malignant, so is it a melanoma or a basal cell carcinoma? Criteria to diagnose a melanocytic lesion are lacking (network, streaks, globules). There are gray-blue blotches throughout the lesion and subtle arborizing vessels (arrow). There are also blue-white structures (asterisks), which should always increase the index of suspicion for a high-risk lesion.

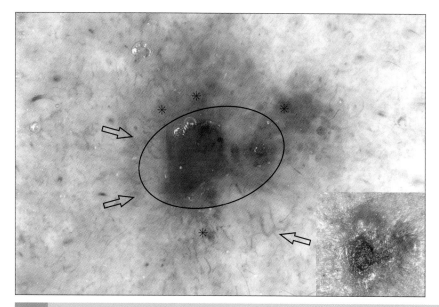

SIX CRITERIA FOR NON-MELANOCYTIC LESIONS

Blue-gray blotches	✔
Arborizing vessels	✔
Milia-like cysts	☐
Comedo-like openings	☐
Red-blue lacunas	☐
Central white patch	☐

Figure 215 Basal cell carcinoma

This small pink lesion has subtle blue-gray blotches, small linear vessels and blue-white structures. Once again the absence of criteria needed to diagnose a melanocytic lesion point towards the dermoscopic diagnosis of a basal cell carcinoma. As long as it is realized that this lesion is not benign, dermoscopy has served its purpose. This is a gray zone lesion.

SIX CRITERIA FOR NON-MELANOCYTIC LESIONS

Blue-gray blotches	✔
Arborizing vessels	✔
Milia-like cysts	☐
Comedo-like openings	☐
Red-blue lacunas	☐
Central white patch	☐

Figure 216 Basal cell carcinoma

Most of this lesion is covered by a crust due to ulceration (circle). There are also small arborizing vessels (arrows) and blue-gray blotches (asterisks). The pigmentation seen in basal cell carcinomas can be brown, gray or blue. It can form well-defined ovoid structures or be indistinct. The more lesions a dermoscopist diagnoses, the better he or she will understand this basic dermoscopic principle. There are numerous variations of all dermoscopic criteria.

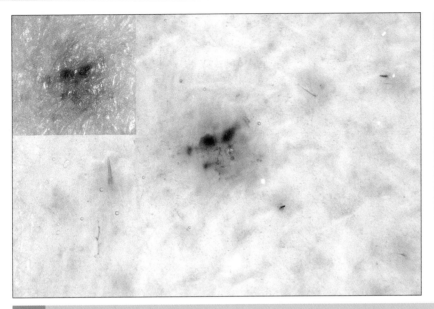

SIX CRITERIA FOR NON-MELANOCYTIC LESIONS

Blue-gray blotches	✔
Arborizing vessels	✔
Milia-like cysts	
Comedo-like openings	
Red-blue lacunas	
Central white patch	

Figure 217 Basal cell carcinoma

Pigmented blotches are the hallmark of this lesion and could be confused with the globules seen in a melanocytic lesion. Some tiny red vessels can also be seen. This is a very non-specific lesion. Other clinical data are needed to make the correct diagnosis.

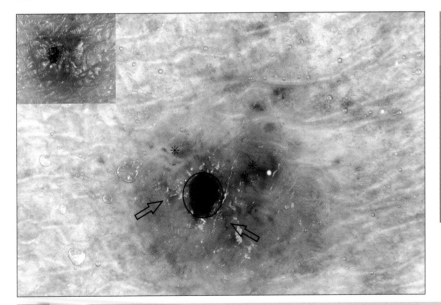

SIX CRITERIA FOR NON-MELANOCYTIC LESIONS

Blue-gray blotches	✔
Arborizing vessels	✔
Milia-like cysts	
Comedo-like openings	
Red-blue lacunas	
Central white patch	

Figure 218 Basal cell carcinoma

Pink lesion – beware. Blue-gray blotches (asterisks), subtle arborizing vessels (arrows) and an area of ulceration (circle) can be seen. These three criteria favor a diagnosis of basal cell carcinoma.

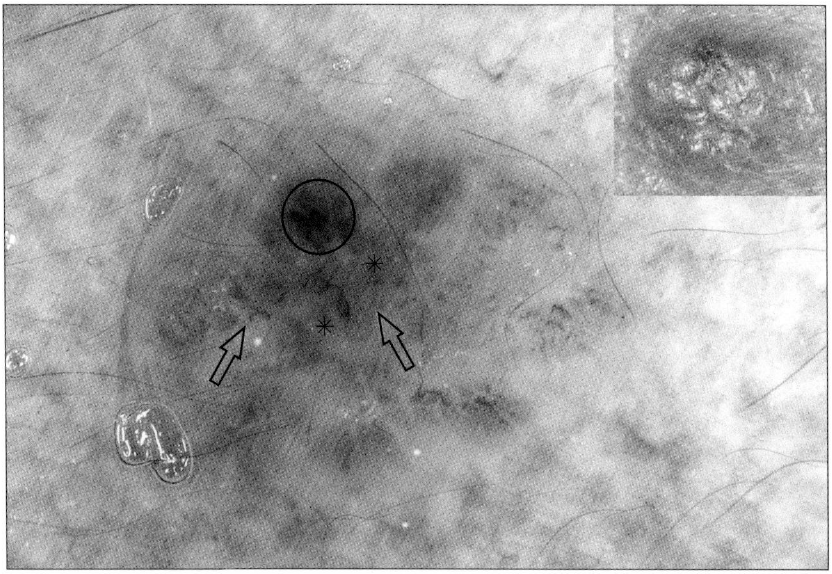

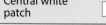

SIX CRITERIA FOR NON-MELANOCYTIC LESIONS	
Blue-gray blotches	✓
Arborizing vessels	✓
Milia-like cysts	☐
Comedo-like openings	☐
Red-blue lacunas	☐
Central white patch	☐

Figure 219 Basal cell carcinoma

This is another basal cell carcinoma with very subtle criteria. On looking closely a blue-gray blotch (asterisks), small arborizing vessels (arrows) and an area of ulceration (circle) can be seen. The light brown color suggests a pigment network, but in reality it is pigmentation in the furrows of this slightly raised papule.

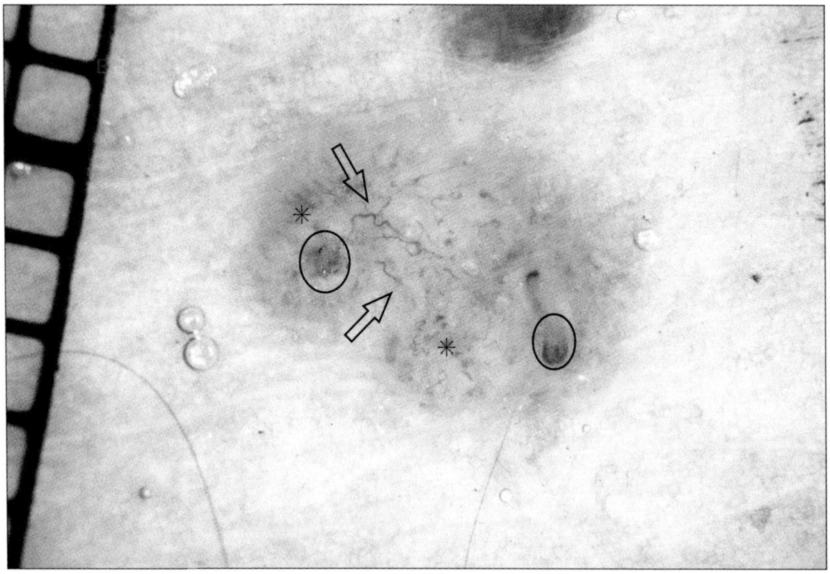

SIX CRITERIA FOR NON-MELANOCYTIC LESIONS	
Blue-gray blotches	✓
Arborizing vessels	✓
Milia-like cysts	☐
Comedo-like openings	☐
Red-blue lacunas	☐
Central white patch	☐

Figure 220 Basal cell carcinoma

The arborizing vessels (arrows) in a clear papule enable diagnosis in this case. There are also subtle blue-gray blotches (asterisks) and areas of ulceration (circles). Important dermoscopic criteria can be easy or difficult to see. Try not to be in a hurry when evaluating a suspicious lesion with dermoscopy.

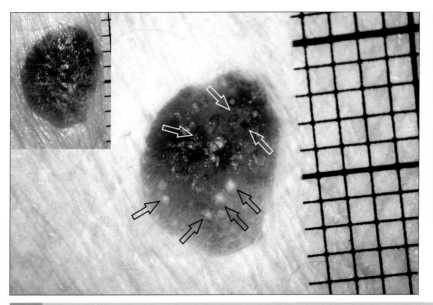

SIX CRITERIA FOR NON-MELANOCYTIC LESIONS	
Blue-gray blotches	☐
Arborizing vessels	☐
Milia-like cysts	☑
Comedo-like openings	☑
Red-blue lacunas	☐
Central white patch	☐

Figure 221 Seborrheic keratosis
The main dermoscopic criteria in this flat plaque are milia-like cysts (black arrows) and comedo-like openings (white arrows), which are diagnostic of a seborrheic keratosis. Using the criteria this is an easy case to diagnose.

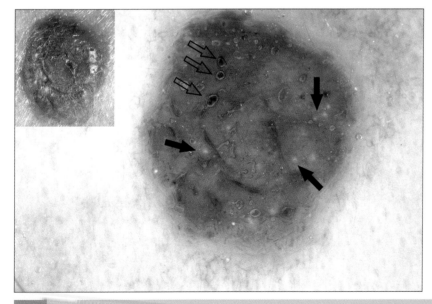

SIX CRITERIA FOR NON-MELANOCYTIC LESIONS	
Blue-gray blotches	☐
Arborizing vessels	☐
Milia-like cysts	☑
Comedo-like openings	☑
Red-blue lacunas	☐
Central white patch	☐

Figure 222 Seborrheic keratosis
In this variant of seborrheic keratosis, comedo-like openings (open arrows) and milia-like cysts (solid arrows) are clearly seen. The dull gray color and the absence of criteria specific for melanocytic lesions argue against the differential diagnosis of a papillomatous melanocytic nevus.

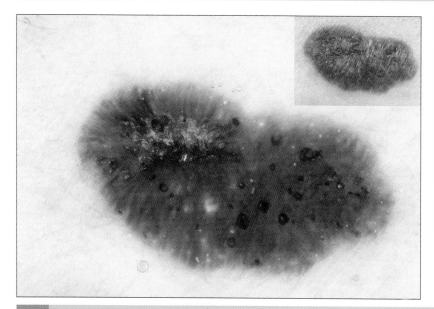

SIX CRITERIA FOR NON-MELANOCYTIC LESIONS	
Blue-gray blotches	☐
Arborizing vessels	☐
Milia-like cysts	☑
Comedo-like openings	☑
Red-blue lacunas	☐
Central white patch	☐

Figure 223 Seborrheic keratosis

This lesion shows good examples of well-developed comedo-like openings (arrows) and a few milia-like cysts. Is there a pigment network in the lower part of the lesion (circle)? No – it is a pseudonetwork formed by the openings of follicles on the face (site-specific criterion). They are not forming the rhomboidal structures of a lentigo maligna.

SIX CRITERIA FOR NON-MELANOCYTIC LESIONS	
Blue-gray blotches	☐
Arborizing vessels	☐
Milia-like cysts	☑
Comedo-like openings	☑
Red-blue lacunas	☐
Central white patch	☐

Figure 224 Seborrheic keratosis

This flat plaque is characterized by multiple comedo-like openings and some milia-like cysts. Looking carefully at the borders of the lesion one might think that there is a starburst pattern of a Spitz nevus. Comedo-like openings and milia-like cysts are as a rule not seen in a Spitz nevus. Perhaps it could be described a pseudostarburst pattern.

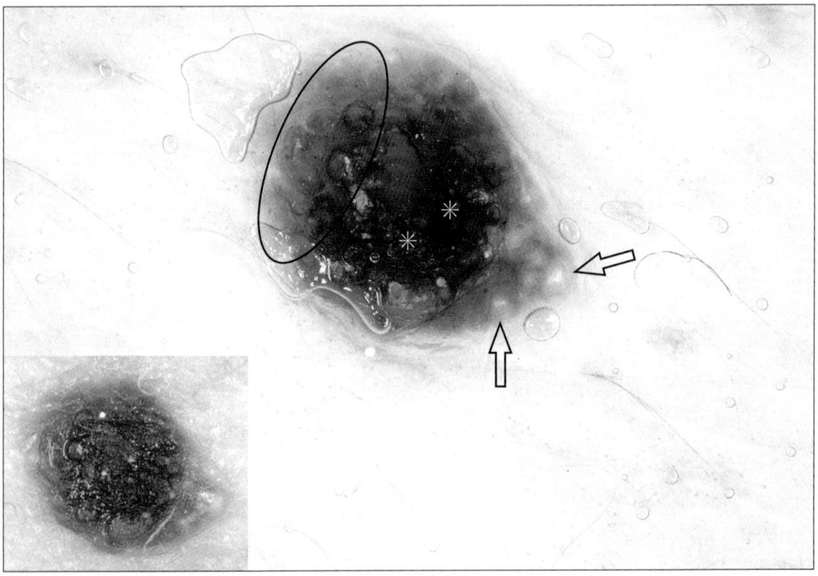

SIX CRITERIA FOR NON-MELANOCYTIC LESIONS

Blue-gray blotches	☐
Arborizing vessels	☐
Milia-like cysts	☑
Comedo-like openings	☐
Red-blue lacunas	☐
Central white patch	☐

Figure 225 Seborrheic keratosis

It is not easy to decide whether this lesion is melanocytic or not. The brown meshes on the left upper part (circle) and central blue-white structures (asterisks) could be interpreted as criteria for a melanocytic lesion. In the lower part, there are milia-like cysts (arrows). If a lesion has asymmetry of color and structure, and the criteria for seborrheic keratosis cannot be clearly recognized, it should be excised. It is better to excise one seborrheic keratosis than miss one melanoma.

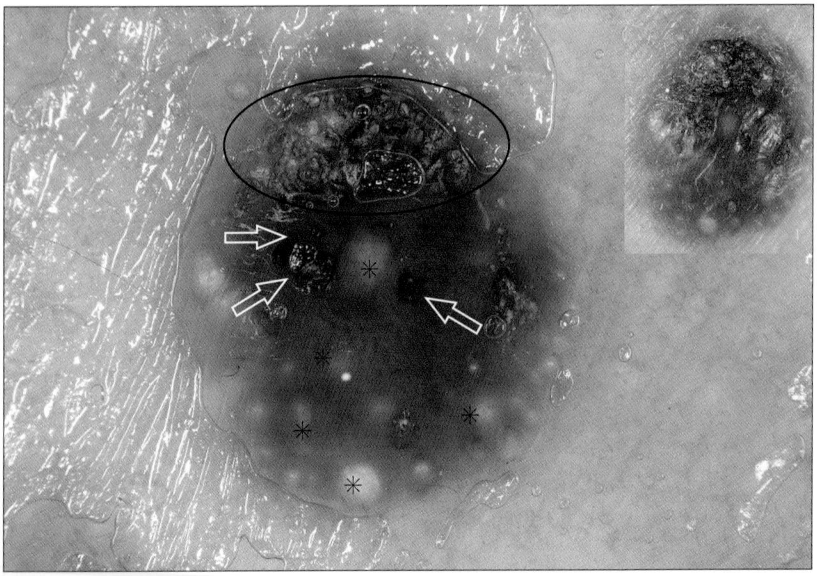

SIX CRITERIA FOR NON-MELANOCYTIC LESIONS

Blue-gray blotches	☐
Arborizing vessels	☐
Milia-like cysts	☑
Comedo-like openings	☑
Red-blue lacunas	☐
Central white patch	☐

Figure 226 Seborrheic keratosis

Opaque color, milia-like cysts (asterisks) and comedo-like openings (arrows) are seen in this lesion with a verrucous surface (circle). This lesion should prove easy to diagnose dermoscopically as a seborrheic keratosis by now.

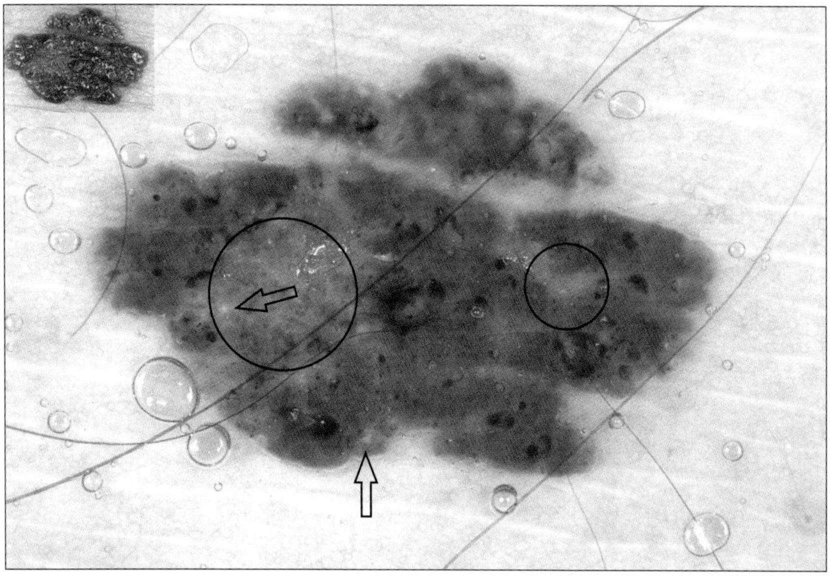

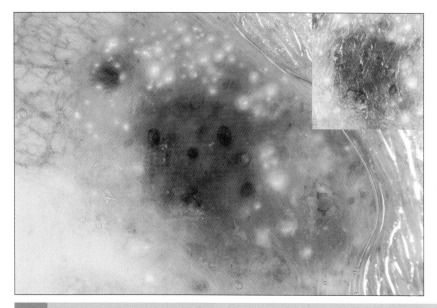

SIX CRITERIA FOR NON-MELANOCYTIC LESIONS	
Blue-gray blotches	☐
Arborizing vessels	☐
Milia-like cysts	☑
Comedo-like openings	☑
Red-blue lacunas	☐
Central white patch	☐

Figure 227 Seborrheic keratosis
Compared to the case shown in Figure 226, this is not so easy to diagnose. This lesion is separated by a few furrows and there are many comedo-like openings. Do not confuse them with the globules of a melanocytic lesion. Subtle milia-like cysts are difficult to find (arrows). There are also hypopigmented areas (circles), which may be seen in seborrheic keratosis. Because of the blue-white structures, this lesion should be excised.

SIX CRITERIA FOR NON-MELANOCYTIC LESIONS	
Blue-gray blotches	☑
Arborizing vessels	☐
Milia-like cysts	☑
Comedo-like openings	☑
Red-blue lacunas	☐
Central white patch	☐

Figure 228 Seborrheic keratosis
A clearcut case of seborrheic keratosis with numerous milia-like cysts and a few comedo-like openings.

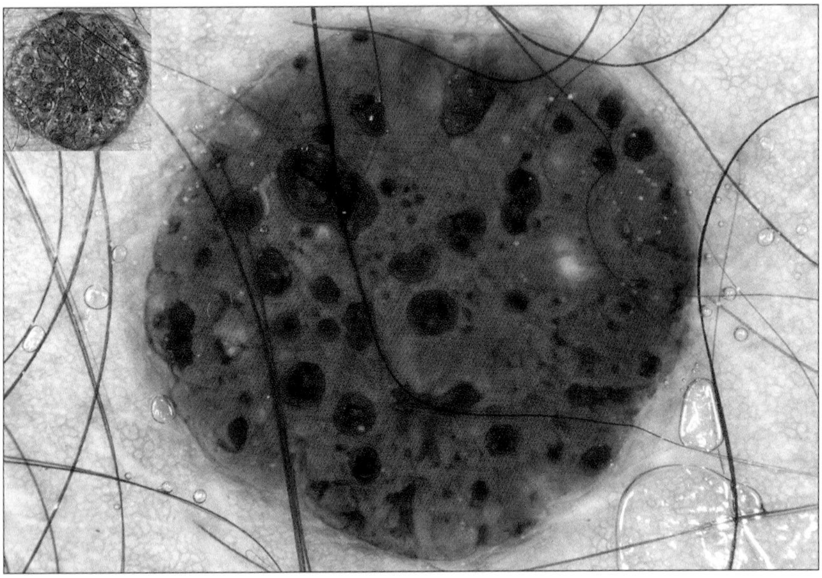

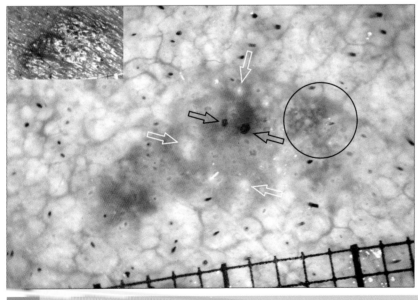

SIX CRITERIA FOR NON-MELANOCYTIC LESIONS	
Blue-gray blotches	☐
Arborizing vessels	☐
Milia-like cysts	☑
Comedo-like openings	☑
Red-blue lacunas	☐
Central white patch	☐

Figure 229 Seborrheic keratosis
This is another stereotypical seborrheic keratosis characterized by numerous comedo-like openings and only a few milia-like cysts. Criteria for a melanocytic lesion are absent.

SIX CRITERIA FOR NON-MELANOCYTIC LESIONS	
Blue-gray blotches	☑
Arborizing vessels	☐
Milia-like cysts	☑
Comedo-like openings	☑
Red-blue lacunas	☐
Central white patch	☐

Figure 230 Seborrheic keratosis
In this flat lesion on the face there are milia-like-cysts (white arrows) and comedo-like openings (black arrows). In one part of the lesion the pigmentation seems to form a pigment network (circle), but this is a pseudopigment network commonly seen on the face. The prominent vessels surrounding the lesion are a common finding in sun-damaged skin.

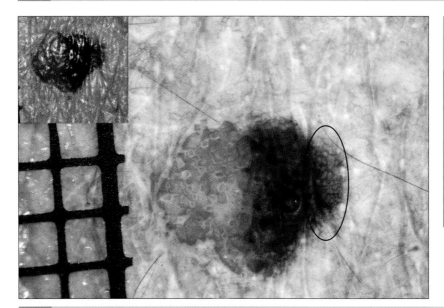

SIX CRITERIA FOR NON-MELANOCYTIC LESIONS	
Blue-gray blotches	☐
Arborizing vessels	☐
Milia-like cysts	☑
Comedo-like openings	☑
Red-blue lacunas	☐
Central white patch	☐

Figure 231 Seborrheic keratosis
Black color and blue-white structures – beware. Remember to look carefully for important criteria to make a dermoscopic diagnosis. This lesion shows multiple milia-like cysts (arrow). It is not possible to determine whether the black color is blotches or comedo-like openings (circles). There is a pronounced verrucous component in the upper part of the lesion, which can be seen in verrucous melanoma. As evidenced by this example, there are many variations of seborrheic keratosis. Remember, when in doubt, cut it out.

SIX CRITERIA FOR NON-MELANOCYTIC LESIONS	
Blue-gray blotches	☑
Arborizing vessels	☐
Milia-like cysts	☐
Comedo-like openings	☑
Red-blue lacunas	☐
Central white patch	☐

Figure 232 Seborrheic keratosis
Despite the striking asymmetry of color and structure, this is a clearcut seborrheic keratosis because there are well-developed comedo-like openings. Is there a pigment network? Are there dots and globules? The network (circle) can rarely be seen in seborrheic keratosis and the dots and gobules are really pigmented comedo-like openings. This is a tricky case that you should not hesitate to excise.

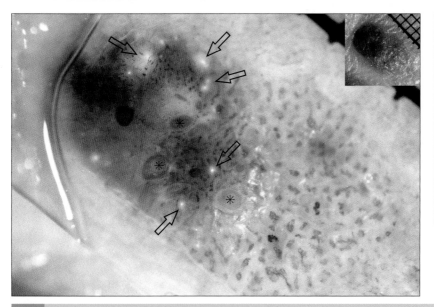

SIX CRITERIA FOR NON-MELANOCYTIC LESIONS

Blue-gray blotches	✓
Arborizing vessels	☐
Milia-like cysts	✓
Comedo-like openings	✓
Red-blue lacunas	☐
Central white patch	☐

Figure 233 Seborrheic keratosis

This unusual seborrheic keratosis is composed of a pigmented area with a grayish color and numerous grayish dots plus a non-pigmented area containing multiple blood vessels. Classic comedo-like openings (asterisks) and milia-like cysts (arrows) lead to the diagnosis. As malignancy can develop in seborrheic keratosis, this lesion should be excised.

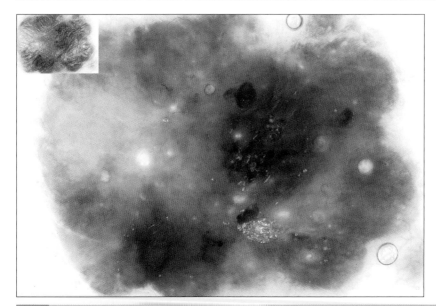

SIX CRITERIA FOR NON-MELANOCYTIC LESIONS

Blue-gray blotches	☐
Arborizing vessels	☐
Milia-like cysts	✓
Comedo-like openings	✓
Red-blue lacunas	☐
Central white patch	☐

Figure 234 Seborrheic keratosis

Despite the striking asymmetry of color and structure and black color, the presence of multiple milia-like cysts and a few comedo-like openings in this lesion is virtually diagnostic of a seborrheic keratosis.

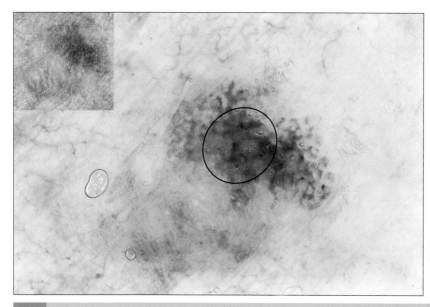

SIX CRITERIA FOR NON-MELANOCYTIC LESIONS	
Blue-gray blotches	✓
Arborizing vessels	☐
Milia-like cysts	✓
Comedo-like openings	✓
Red-blue lacunas	☐
Central white patch	☐

Figure 235 Seborrheic keratosis

This is a seborrheic keratosis localized on the face and characterized by comedo-like openings (white arrows) and a few tiny milia-like cysts (black arrows). The grayish color can be seen in irritated and regressive lesions. The blue-gray blotches (circles) could increase one's index of suspicion of a high-risk lesion. If in doubt, cut it out! We cannnot overemphasize this basic dermoscopic principle.

SIX CRITERIA FOR NON-MELANOCYTIC LESIONS	
Blue-gray blotches	☐
Arborizing vessels	☐
Milia-like cysts	☐
Comedo-like openings	☐
Red-blue lacunas	☐
Central white patch	☐

Figure 236 Seborrheic keratosis

This is a very unusual seborrheic keratosis with an atypical pigment network in the right upper section of the lesion. There are no clear criteria to diagnose a seborrheic keratosis and there is a suggestion of the rhomboidal structures (circle) that are seen in lentigo maligna. This lesion should therefore be excised.

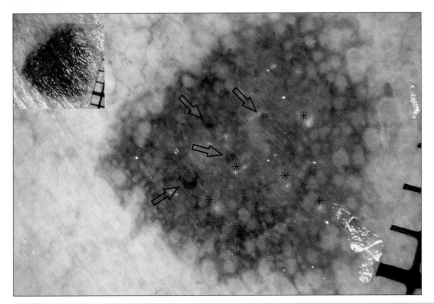

SIX CRITERIA FOR NON-MELANOCYTIC LESIONS

Blue-gray blotches	☐
Arborizing vessels	☐
Milia-like cysts	☑
Comedo-like openings	☑
Red-blue lacunas	☐
Central white patch	☐

Figure 237 Seborrheic keratosis
This is another example of seborrheic keratosis on the face characterized by a brownish-gray pseudoreticular pattern simulating lentigo maligna. The diagnosis of a seborrheic keratosis is suggested because there are a few milia-like cysts (asterisks) and comedo-like openings (arrows). This is another difficult case to diagnose, of which unfortunately there are many. Always err on the side of caution and excise equivocal lesions with a confusing dermoscopic picture.

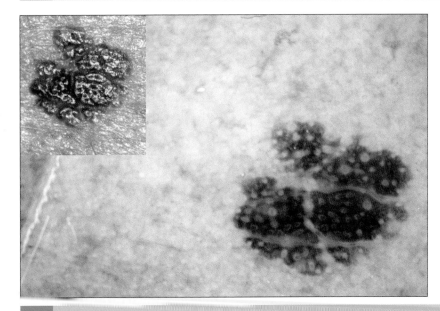

SIX CRITERIA FOR NON-MELANOCYTIC LESIONS

Blue-gray blotches	☐
Arborizing vessels	☐
Milia-like cysts	☐
Comedo-like openings	☑
Red-blue lacunas	☐
Central white patch	☐

Figure 238 Seborrheic keratosis
This shows yet another variation of the morphology seen in seborrheic keratosis located on the face. Are the multiple light-yellow circles comedo-like openings or follicular openings? It is hard to make the differentiation, but we favor comedo-like openings. Clinically, it looks like a seborrheic keratosis, and with dermoscopy there are no high-risk criteria suggestive of lentigo maligna.

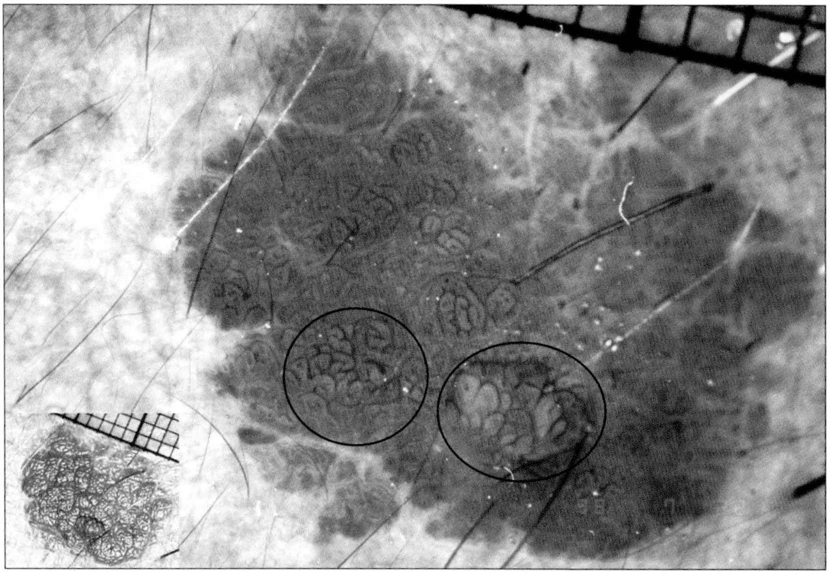

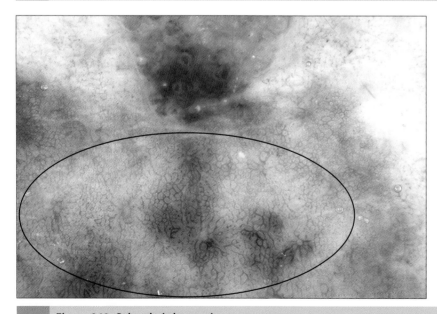

SIX CRITERIA FOR NON-MELANOCYTIC LESIONS

Blue-gray blotches	☐
Arborizing vessels	☐
Milia-like cysts	☐
Comedo-like openings	☐
Red-blue lacunas	☐
Central white patch	☐

Figure 239 Seborrheic keratosis
This seborrheic keratosis with a brain-like pattern displays fissures and ridges (circles) mimicking the gyri and sulci of the brain. The brain-like pattern is diagnostic of seborrheic keratosis.

SIX CRITERIA FOR NON-MELANOCYTIC LESIONS

Blue-gray blotches	☐
Arborizing vessels	☐
Milia-like cysts	☑
Comedo-like openings	☑
Red-blue lacunas	☐
Central white patch	☐

Figure 240 Seborrheic keratosis
This is a collision lesion – two different pathologies in one. A banal melanocytic lesion is represented by the typical pigment network (circle) and a seborrheic keratosis has a few milia-like cysts and comedo-like openings. As there is asymmetry of color and structure, a histopathologic diagnosis is recommended.

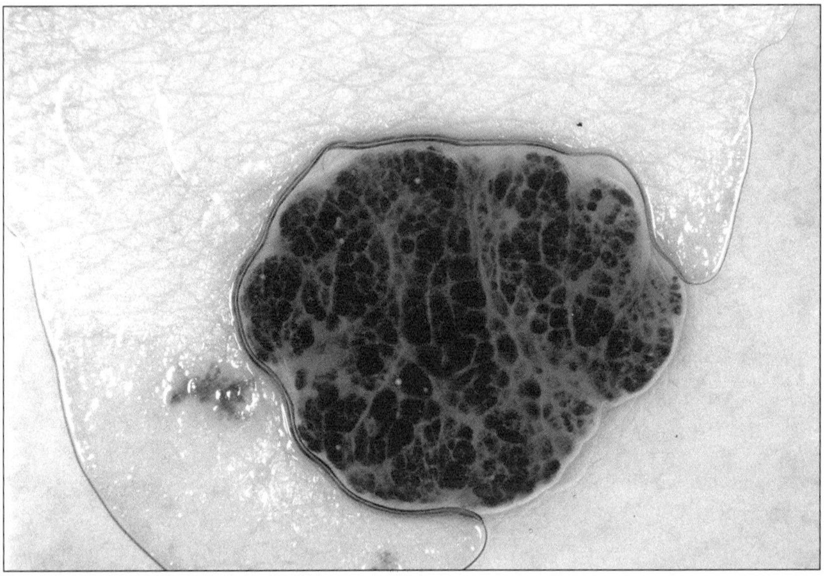

SIX CRITERIA FOR NON-MELANOCYTIC LESIONS	
Blue-gray blotches	☐
Arborizing vessels	☐
Milia-like cysts	☐
Comedo-like openings	☐
Red-blue lacunas	☑
Central white patch	☐

Figure 241 Hemangioma

This is a classic hemangioma with multiple red lacunas. They are well-demarcated, reddish, round-to-polygonal structures that correspond to the dilated vessels in the upper dermis. White color is commonly found in hemangiomas; in this case it has a reticular pattern. There is no doubt of the dermoscopic diagnosis in this case.

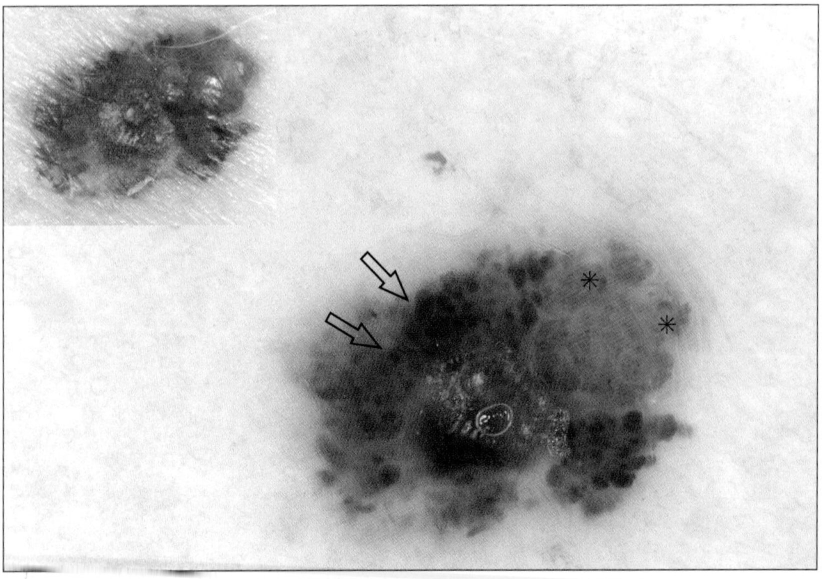

SIX CRITERIA FOR NON-MELANOCYTIC LESIONS	
Blue-gray blotches	☐
Arborizing vessels	☐
Milia-like cysts	☐
Comedo-like openings	☐
Red-blue lacunas	☑
Central white patch	☐

Figure 242 Hemangioma

This vascular lesion is characterized by red (asterisks) and purplish (arrows) lacunas. It is possible to confuse the blue-to-purplish color with a blue-white structure. It is unusual to find two colors in a hemangioma. If in doubt, cut it out.

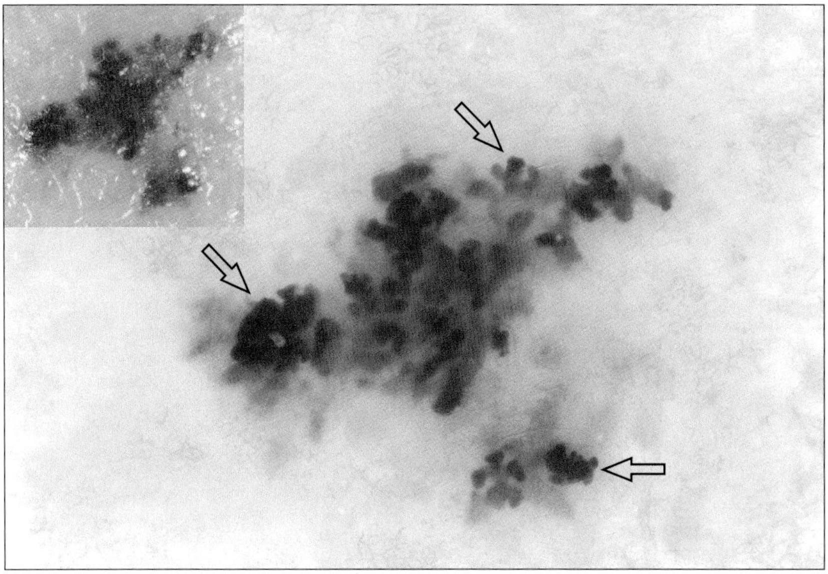

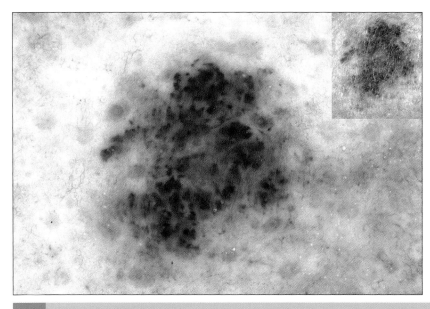

SIX CRITERIA FOR NON-MELANOCYTIC LESIONS

Blue-gray blotches	☐
Arborizing vessels	☐
Milia-like cysts	☐
Comedo-like openings	☐
Red-blue lacunas	☑
Central white patch	☐

Figure 243 Hemangioma

This is another stereotypical example of cherry (senile) hemangioma and has numerous well-circumscribed red-blue lacunas (arrows).

Remember that to diagnose the lacunas they should have sharp borders. The should be clear and not out of focus or blurred.

SIX CRITERIA FOR NON-MELANOCYTIC LESIONS

Blue-gray blotches	☐
Arborizing vessels	☐
Milia-like cysts	☐
Comedo-like openings	☐
Red-blue lacunas	☑
Central white patch	☐

Figure 244 Hemangioma

This hemangioma displays a diffuse blue-white color that mimicks blue-white structures. Closer scrutiny reveals multiple well-developed lacunas filling the lesion.

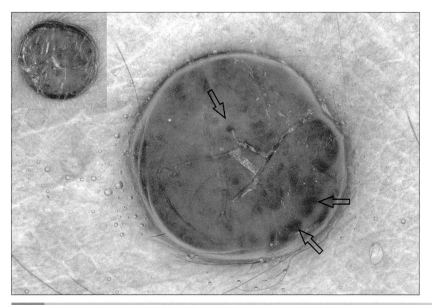

SIX CRITERIA FOR NON-MELANOCYTIC LESIONS	
Blue-gray blotches	☐
Arborizing vessels	☐
Milia-like cysts	☐
Comedo-like openings	☐
Red-blue lacunas	✔
Central white patch	☐

Figure 245 Fibroangioma

This is a fibroangioma characterized by a diffuse reddish color, which is the hallmark of the lesion. There are a few subtle red lacunas (arrows) and the diffuse white color represents fibrosis. Pyogenic granuloma, Kaposi´s sarcoma and amelanotic melanoma could have a similar dermoscopic appearance.

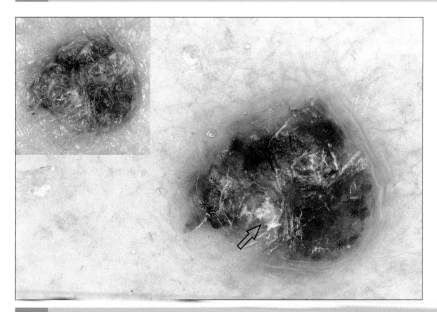

SIX CRITERIA FOR NON-MELANOCYTIC LESIONS	
Blue-gray blotches	☐
Arborizing vessels	☐
Milia-like cysts	☐
Comedo-like openings	☐
Red-blue lacunas	✔
Central white patch	☐

Figure 246 Angiokeratoma

This is an example of angiokeratoma characterized by red-blue lacunas (asterisks) and whitish scaly areas (arrow) that represent hyperkeratosis. The combination of red-blue color with a scaly surface is the dermoscopic hallmark of an angiokeratoma. Quite often, angiokeratomas mimic melanoma clinically; dermoscopy is very helpful in making the correct diagnosis.

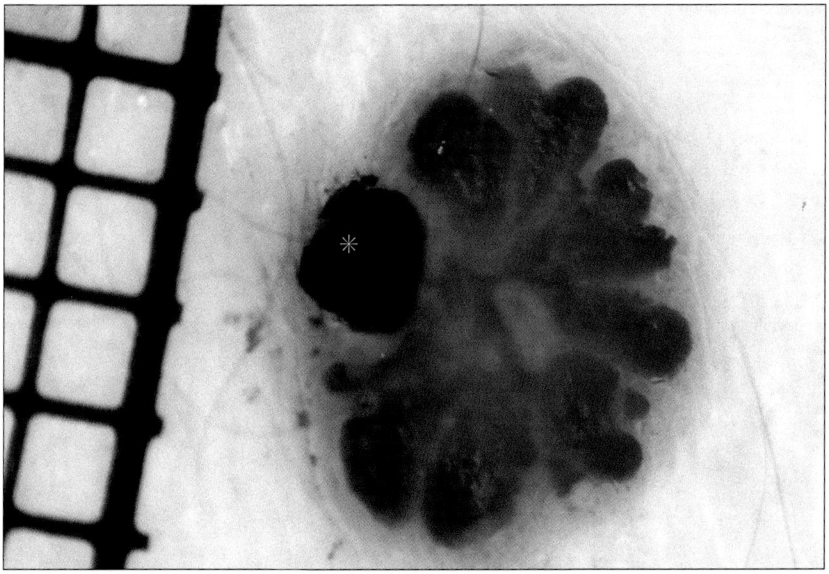

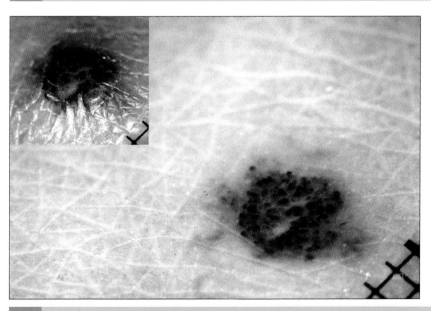

SIX CRITERIA FOR
NON-MELANOCYTIC
LESIONS

Blue-gray blotches	☐
Arborizing vessels	☐
Milia-like cysts	☐
Comedo-like openings	☐
Red-blue lacunas	☑
Central white patch	☐

Figure 247 Hemangioma
This hemangioma is partially thrombosed. The reddish-black areas represent thrombosed vascular spaces (asterisk) and not the blotches of a melanoma.

SIX CRITERIA FOR
NON-MELANOCYTIC
LESIONS

Blue-gray blotches	☐
Arborizing vessels	☐
Milia-like cysts	☐
Comedo-like openings	☐
Red-blue lacunas	☑
Central white patch	☐

Figure 248 Hemangioma
This hemangioma is characterized by red-blue lacunas with a predominantly bluish color. The peripheral light-blue halo indicates deeper involvement of the hemangioma in the dermis.

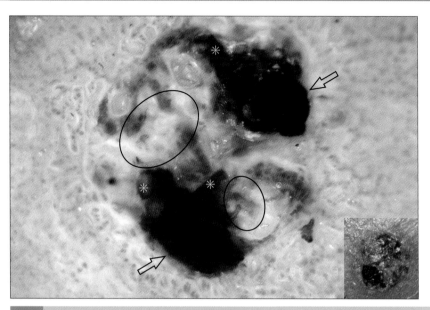

SIX CRITERIA FOR NON-MELANOCYTIC LESIONS

Blue-gray blotches	✔
Arborizing vessels	☐
Milia-like cysts	☐
Comedo-like openings	☐
Red-blue lacunas	✔
Central white patch	☐

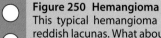

Figure 249 Hemangioma

The gray-black blotches and white color are worrisome criteria even for the experienced dermoscopist. However, this is another example of a thrombosed hemangioma. It has red-blue (asterisks) to red-black (arrows) lacunas corresponding to the thrombosed areas. The whitish color (circles) represents fibrosis in the dermis. Excision of a lesion that looks like this is indicated.

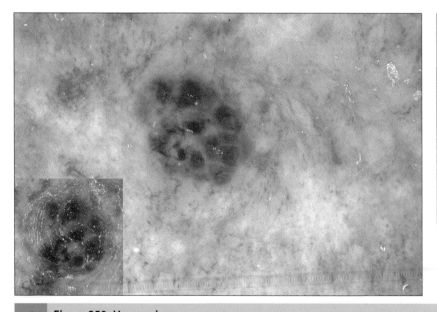

SIX CRITERIA FOR NON-MELANOCYTIC LESIONS

Blue-gray blotches	☐
Arborizing vessels	☐
Milia-like cysts	☐
Comedo-like openings	☐
Red-blue lacunas	✔
Central white patch	☐

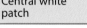

Figure 250 Hemangioma

This typical hemangioma displays well-developed reddish lacunas. What about the pinkish-white color adjacent to the lesion? Could this be regressive melanoma that happens to be next to the ubiquitous hemangioma, or just severely sun-damaged skin?

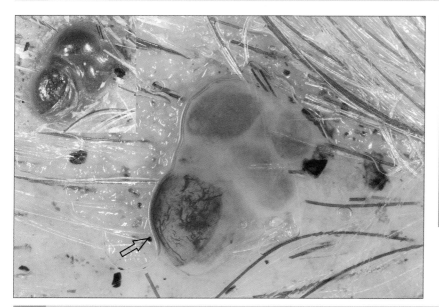

SIX CRITERIA FOR NON-MELANOCYTIC LESIONS

Blue-gray blotches	☐
Arborizing vessels	☐
Milia-like cysts	☐
Comedo-like openings	☐
Red-blue lacunas	✓
Central white patch	☐

Figure 251 Hemangioma

This shows a variation of the morphology that can be seen with a partially thrombosed hemangioma. It is characterized by large red-blue to red-black lacunas. The reddish color on the left (circle) represents a traumatized hemorrhagic area. There are many faces of vascular lesions. The red-to-purplish color is key to making the diagnosis. But remember, if in doubt, cut it out.

SIX CRITERIA FOR NON-MELANOCYTIC LESIONS

Blue-gray blotches	☐
Arborizing vessels	☐
Milia-like cysts	☐
Comedo-like openings	☐
Red-blue lacunas	✓
Central white patch	☐

Figure 252 Pyogenic granuloma

This is a vascular lesion because it has large red lacunas. Numerous telangiectasias are also present (arrow). The diagnosis of a pyogenic granuloma can be made only on clinical or histopathologic grounds because precise differentiation from a hemangioma is not possible with dermoscopy. Remember that amelanotic melanoma, the great masquerader, is always in the differential diagnosis of a pyogenic granuloma.

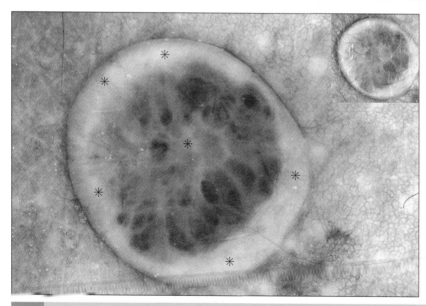

SIX CRITERIA FOR NON-MELANOCYTIC LESIONS	
Blue-gray blotches	☐
Arborizing vessels	☐
Milia-like cysts	☐
Comedo-like openings	☐
Red-blue lacunas	☑
Central white patch	☐

Figure 253 Kaposi´s sarcoma

The dermoscopic appearance of this vascular nodule is non-specific and is similar to the pyogenic granuloma and the fibroangioma shown in Figure 245. There are red lacunas and whitish areas of fibrosis (asterisks). Important historical and clinical data might be needed to help diagnose certain vascular-appearing lesions.

SIX CRITERIA FOR NON-MELANOCYTIC LESIONS	
Blue-gray blotches	☐
Arborizing vessels	☐
Milia-like cysts	☐
Comedo-like openings	☐
Red-blue lacunas	☑
Central white patch	☐

Figure 254 Hemangioma

As in the previous figures, this vascular lesion exhibits red lacunas with pronounced whitish areas of fibrosis (asterisks). The dermoscopic differential diagnosis includes fibroangioma and fibrosing pyogenic granuloma. As a rule, the dermoscopic aspect of a lesion should be part of the overall clinical assessment of the patient. This is another basic dermoscopic principle that cannot be overemphasized.

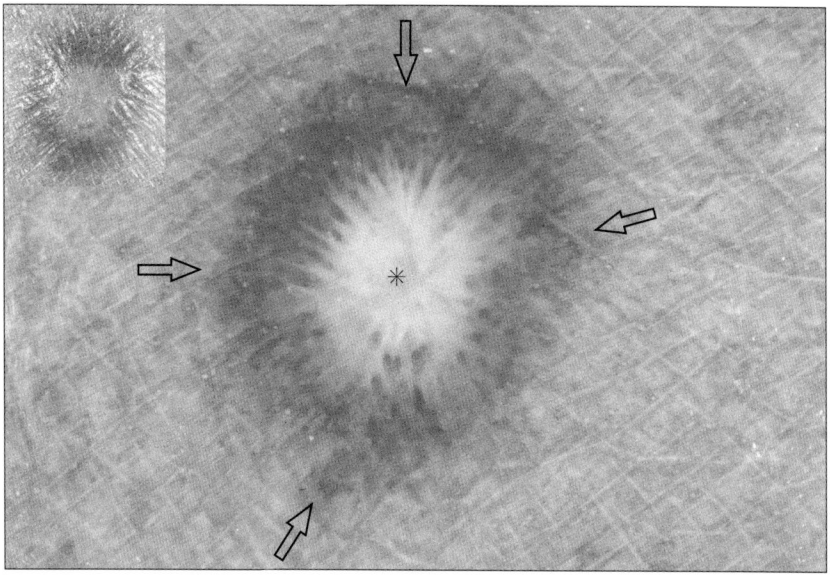

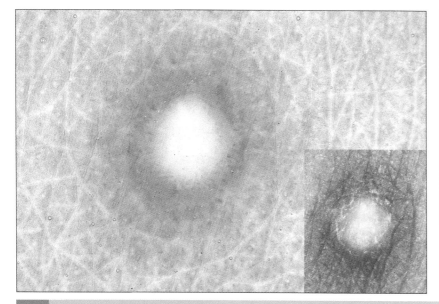

SIX CRITERIA FOR NON-MELANOCYTIC LESIONS	
Blue-gray blotches	☐
Arborizing vessels	☐
Milia-like cysts	☐
Comedo-like openings	☐
Red-blue lacunas	☐
Central white patch	☑

Figure 255 Dermatofibroma

This stereotypical dermatofibroma with a central white patch (asterisk) is surrounded by a very subtle pigment network (arrows). Dermatofibromas are one of the few non-melanocytic lesions that can have a pigment network.

SIX CRITERIA FOR NON-MELANOCYTIC LESIONS	
Blue-gray blotches	☐
Arborizing vessels	☐
Milia-like cysts	☐
Comedo-like openings	☐
Red-blue lacunas	☐
Central white patch	☑

Figure 256 Dermatofibroma

In this dermatofibroma the central white patch predominates. Light pigmentation, but not a network, can be seen at the periphery. Palpating this firm papule will help in making the diagnosis. There are numerous variations of the white patch seen in dermatofibromas.

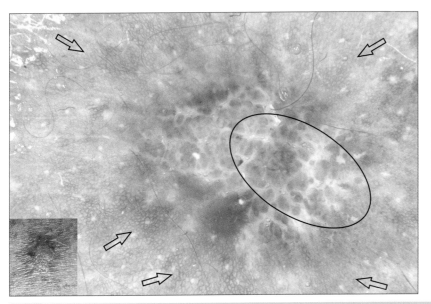

SIX CRITERIA FOR NON-MELANOCYTIC LESIONS	
Blue-gray blotches	☐
Arborizing vessels	☐
Milia-like cysts	☐
Comedo-like openings	☐
Red-blue lacunas	☐
Central white patch	✔

Figure 257 Dermatofibroma
This dermatofibroma has a reticular depigmentation (circle), which is a variation of the central white patch. A very subtle pigment network can also be seen at the periphery (arrows). A reticular white color is commonly seen in dermatofibromas.

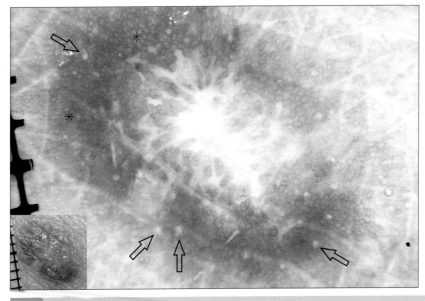

SIX CRITERIA FOR NON-MELANOCYTIC LESIONS	
Blue-gray blotches	☐
Arborizing vessels	☐
Milia-like cysts	✔
Comedo-like openings	☐
Red-blue lacunas	☐
Central white patch	✔

Figure 258 Dermatofibroma
This is another example of classic dermatofibroma with a central white patch and a fine typical pigment network at the periphery (asterisks). Do not diagnose this as seborrheic keratosis because milia-like cysts (arrows) can be seen.

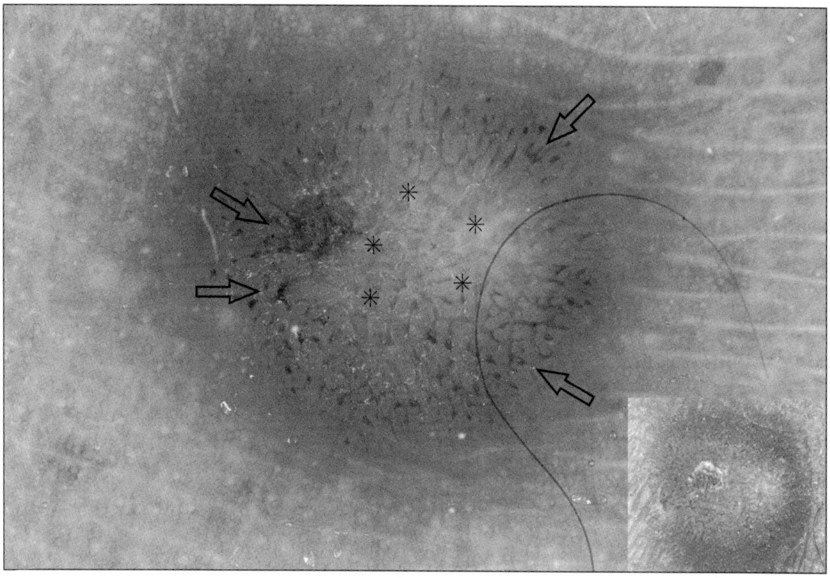

SIX CRITERIA FOR NON-MELANOCYTIC LESIONS	
Blue-gray blotches	☐
Arborizing vessels	☐
Milia-like cysts	☐
Comedo-like openings	☐
Red-blue lacunas	☐
Central white patch	☑

Figure 259 Dermatofibroma

This dermatofibroma has a central white patch (asterisks) and barely detectable pigment network at the periphery. There are also multiple dots and globules and pigmented streaks (arrows), which represent pigmentation in the fissures of a raised lesion. Do not confuse them with the criteria for diagnosing other pigmented lesions. Any verrucous neoplasm, regardless of the pathology, melanocytic or non-melanocytic, may have pigmented fissures.

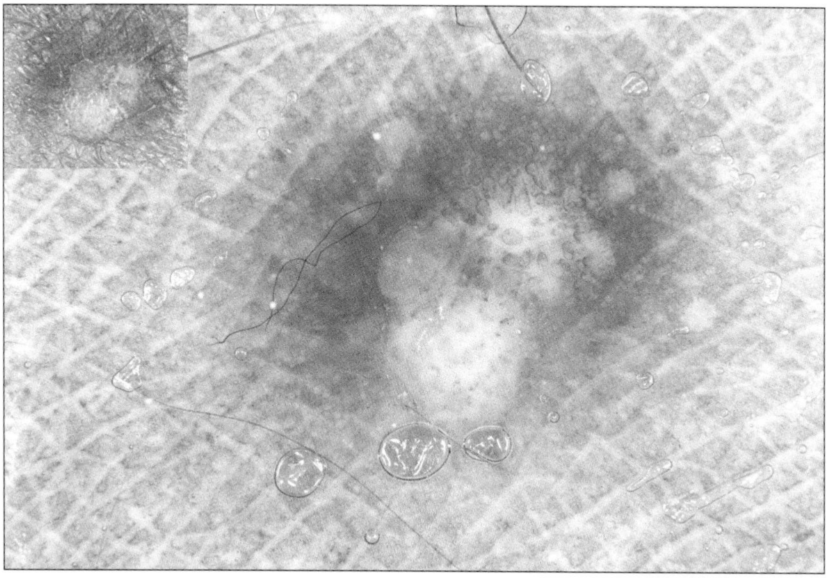

SIX CRITERIA FOR NON-MELANOCYTIC LESIONS	
Blue-gray blotches	☐
Arborizing vessels	☐
Milia-like cysts	☐
Comedo-like openings	☐
Red-blue lacunas	☐
Central white patch	☑

Figure 260 Dermatofibroma

Here is another dermatofibroma illustrating the many faces of the central white patch.

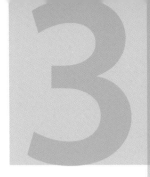

Common Clinical Scenarios

Side-by-side comparisons of similar appearing lesions that are benign or malignant

INTRODUCTION

When you examine a skin lesion with dermoscopy it might be obviously benign or malignant. There is also a gray zone of equivocal lesions. Gray zone lesions will commonly be encountered by the novice dermoscopist. To help deal with this common situation, we offer a few suggestions. Learn the basics, practice the technique as often as possible, and develop a dermoscopic differential diagnosis.

You have to be able to think things through logically, weighing the pros and cons for each criterion or pattern that you see. Coming up with a tentative dermoscopic diagnosis, or in many cases a dermoscopic differential diagnosis, is the end of the process.

For example, are the round to oval yellow dots and globules you see the milia-like cysts of a seborrheic keratosis, or the follicular ostia of a melanocytic lesion? What a difference that distinction could make. You could be dealing with a seborrheic keratosis or a lentigo maligna. Are those the brown dots and globules of a melanocytic lesion, or the pigmented follicular openings of a seborrheic keratosis? You notice that the lesion has some blood vessels. Are they the thickened branched vessels of a basal cell carcinoma, or the irregular linear vessels that can be found in melanomas?

We regret to inform you that you will encounter difficult lesions – lesions that even the most experienced dermoscopist will not feel confident with. That is the state of the art as it exists today. There are infinite variations of criteria, patterns and lesions. The scenarios in this final chapter demonstrate the dermoscopic thought process we employ. Focus your attention, use what you have learned in the first two chapters of the book and you will find that you will learn and grow with each case. Do not be intimidated by what you see. We guarantee that you can master this technique. You will develop your own style of dermoscopic analysis and find that dermoscopy will become an essential part of your practice. You won't be able to practice without it!

PEDIATRIC SCENARIO

GENERAL PRINCIPLES

- No pediatric patient (20 years of age or younger) should have a pigmented skin lesion biopsied or excised before being examined with dermoscopy. The frequency of dysplastic nevi or melanoma is very low in this age group and unnecessary operations can be avoided.
- Dermoscopic criteria are the same in all age groups.

- A pigmented skin lesion that looks high risk in a pediatric patient both clinically or with dermoscopy is high risk until proven otherwise. Make the diagnosis sooner rather than later.
- Relatively featureless and amelanotic dysplastic nevi and melanomas can be seen in the pediatric population.

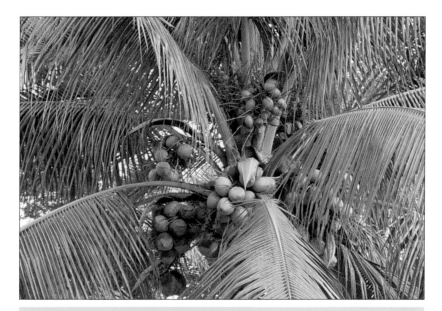

You can relax under these globules, and you can relax if you see them in a pigmented skin lesion, because they are uniform in size and shape.

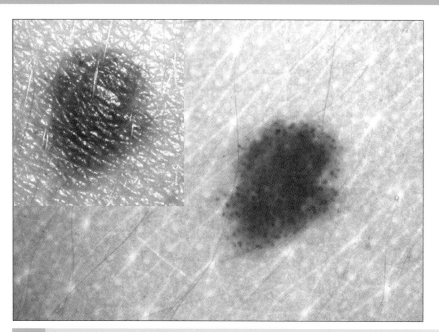

Figure 261 Clark (dysplastic) nevus

This is one example of the three moderately dysplastic nevi diagnosed in a 5-year-old child with skin phototype II. Two lesions were on the back and one was hidden in the scalp. None of the nevi demonstrated the clinical ABCDs, but with dermoscopy there was asymmetry of irregular dots and globules.

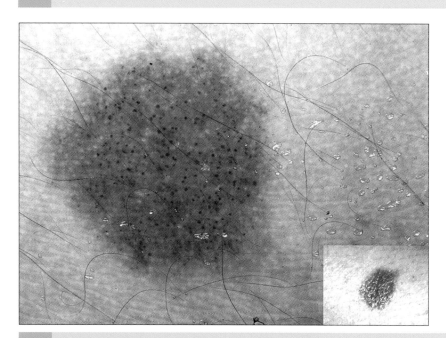

Figure 262 Nevus

A 3-year-old child was being evaluated before surgery to remove a giant congenital melanocytic nevus on the scalp. The patient's mother stated that the surgeon was going to excise a nevus on her leg too because the child would be under general anesthesia anyway. Clinically and with dermoscopy the nevus on her leg was considered to be low risk with a globular pattern. Based on this dermoscopic picture, an unnecessary excision was avoided, decreasing the time under general anesthesia.

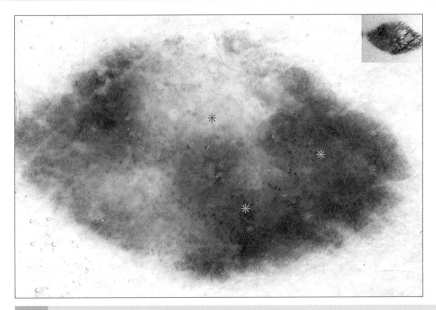

Figure 263 Spitz nevus

At any age this is a very worrisome dermoscopic picture. There is a multicomponent global pattern, asymmetry of color and structure with two melanoma-specific criteria – a white blue-white structure (black asterisk) and irregular dots and globules (white asterisks). Also notice the pink color. Although this patient was young, when the pathology report came back showing this to be a Spitz nevus we asked for a second opinion to rule out melanoma.

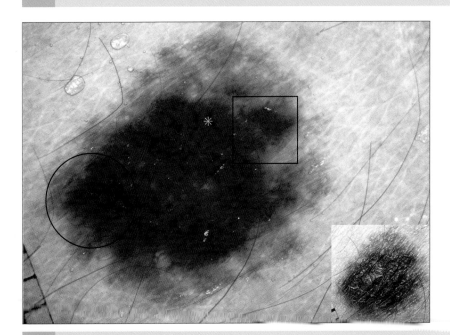

Figure 264 Clark (dysplastic) nevus

This is another very worrisome lesion that happens to be in a young patient. It contains several melanoma-specific criteria – a dark blotch (white asterisk), a blue-white structure (black asterisk), irregular streaks (circle) and a subtle atypical pigment network (square). Black color is not pathognomonic of melanoma in any age group. The worst-looking dermoscopic picture might not be melanoma. Never tell your patient that it is 100% certain that they have a melanoma.

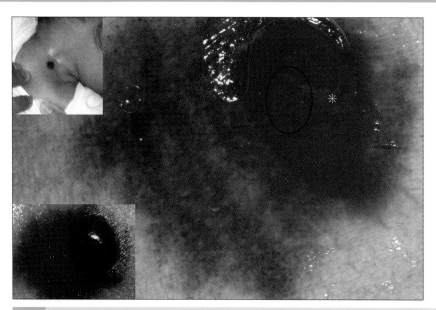

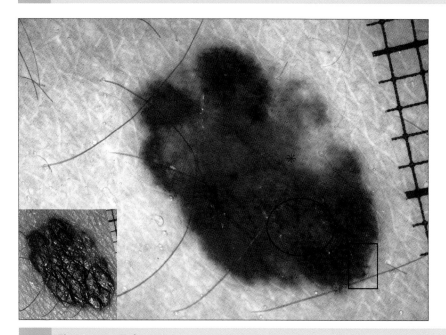

Figure 265 Congenital melanoma

This was a rapidly growing nodule in a small congenital melanocytic nevus present at birth. With dermoscopy there was a blue-white structure (asterisk) and black dots (circle). The dilemma was not whether it needed to be excised, but when. The surgeon wanted to wait until the patient was 6 months old because general anesthesia would be safer. Based on the high-risk dermoscopic picture we recommend excision as soon as possible.

Figure 266 Melanoma

This is a melanoma on a 14-year-old child. It has melanoma-specific criteria – a blue-white structure (asterisk), which is easy to see, subtle streaks (square) and irregular dots and globules (circle). Young patients do get melanoma and die from their disease, so it is necessary to increase one's index of suspicion for pediatric patients.

ACRAL LESIONS

GENERAL PRINCIPLES

- Asymmetry of color and structure – rule out melanoma.
- Parallel ridge pattern = melanoma.
- Parallel furrow, lattice, fibrillar patterns = benign lesions.
- Purple color = blood.
- Blood can be found in nail apparatus and acral lentiginous melanomas; therefore if blood is seen search for melanoma-specific criteria.
- Most importantly, if in doubt, cut it out.

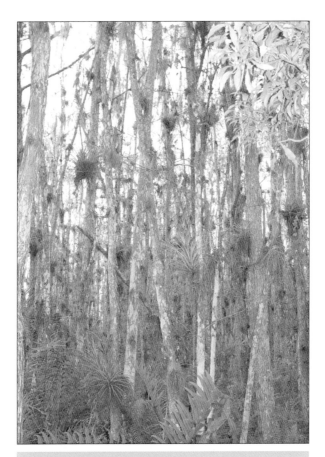

These are parallel, aren't they?

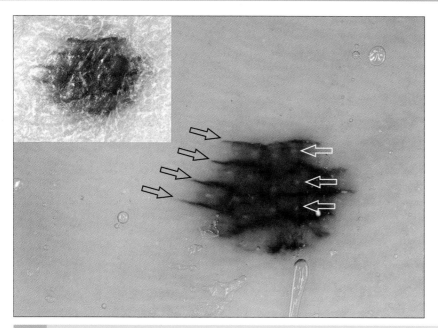

Figure 267 Nevus

Parallel ridge? Parallel furrow? The linear darker brown color is pigmentation in the furrows (black arrows). White dots, the 'string of pearls' (white arrows), are always in the ridges. There is also a blue-white structure (asterisk). Err on the side of caution and do a biopsy, and the dermoscopist will feel more confident the next time he or she sees a nevus that looks like this.

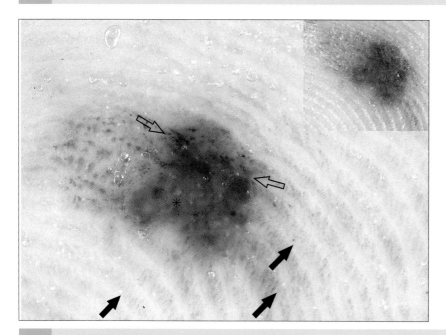

Figure 268 Melanoma

This lesion shows the parallel ridge pattern (solid arrows). There is also asymmetry of color and structure, atypical dots and globules (open arrows) and a blue-white structure (asterisk). This is a melanoma until proven otherwise.

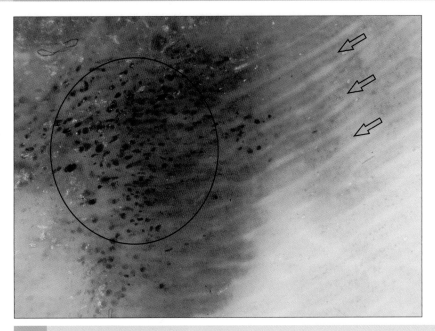

Figure 269 Melanoma

Parallel ridge? Parallel furrow? The 'string of pearls' white dots of the sweat duct pores cannot be seen clearly, but this is the high-risk parallel ridge (arrows) pattern. If the dermoscopist is not sure what to do, the irregular dots and globules (circle) are worrisome enough by themselves to warrant a biopsy.

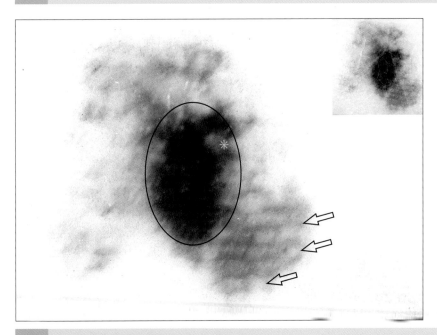

Figure 270 Melanoma

Parallel ridge? Parallel furrow? Does this look like the parallel furrow pattern of a benign nevus? The irregular dark blotch (circle) and blue-white structure (asterisk) reveal that this is melanoma, and it is arising in a nevus with a parallel furrow pattern (arrows).

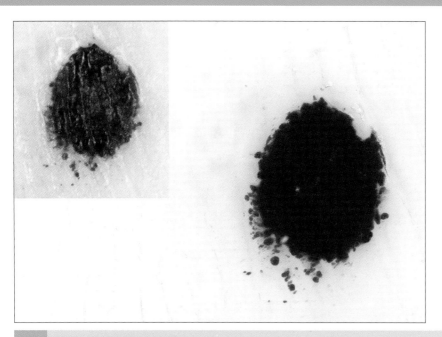

Figure 271 Subcorneal hemorrhage

Is the color here black or purple? It is purplish and amorphous (structureless), therefore it is blood. Take a needle and poke some out. Needling is a simple test to confirm that one is dealing with blood. Another clue that this is blood is the purplish dots adjacent to the lesion.

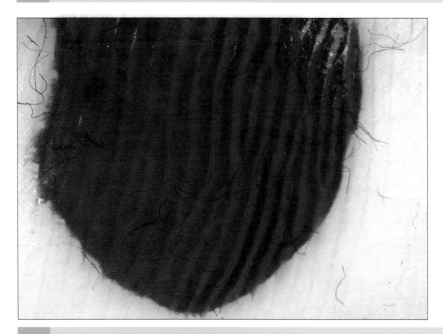

Figure 272 Subcorneal hemorrhage

This is the color of blood, but with a pattern. Parallel ridge? Parallel furrow? Check the surrounding skin. Ridges are thicker than furrows. The blood is in both. The ridges are the darker lines. If unconvinced, needle out some of the dried blood. Pink skin should be seen where the blood was.

BLACK LESIONS

GENERAL PRINCIPLES

- Clinically, black color is not always ominous.
- Black color with dermoscopy is not always ominous.
- The differential diagnosis of a single black macule or papule could be melanocytic, non-melanocytic, benign or malignant.

- What should be done on finding a black lesion? Check it out with dermoscopy before making another move.

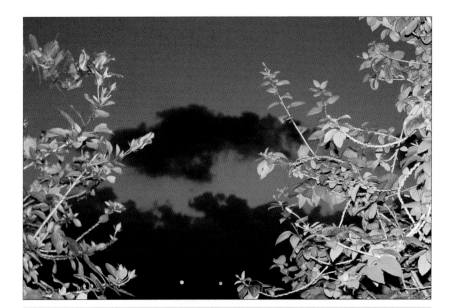

The irregular black clouds of an impending summer storm look remarkably similar to the irregular black blotches in another impending storm, melanoma.

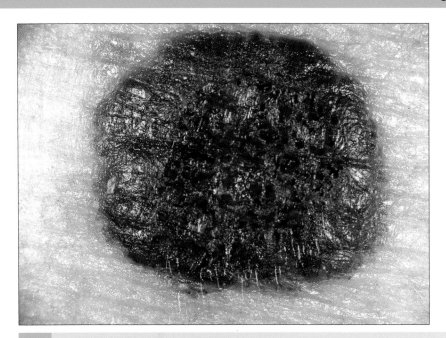

Figure 273 What is your clinical diagnosis?
This clinically non-specific black lesion looks like that in Figure 274. There is no way to know for sure which is benign and which is malignant. What should be done? Cut it out or check it out (see Figure 275)?

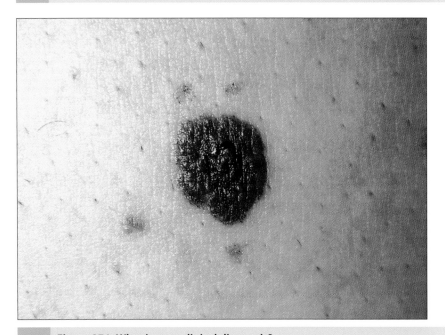

Figure 274 What is your clinical diagnosis?
This clinically non-specific black lesion looks like that in Figure 273. There is no way to know for sure which is benign and which is malignant. What should be done? Cut it out or check it out (see Figure 276)?

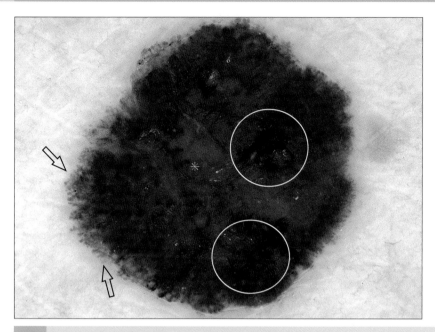

Figure 275 Melanoma
Step one – is it melanocytic or non-melanocytic? It is a melanocytic lesion because there are streaks at the periphery (arrows). Step 2 – is it benign or malignant? Can melanoma-specific criteria be identified? The blue-white structure (asterisk) and irregular blotches (circles) are enough to warrant excision as soon as possible.

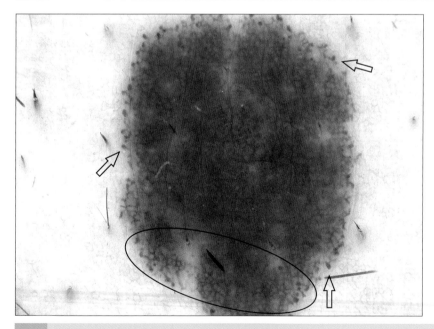

Figure 276 Nevus
A sigh of relief. This is a benign nevus because of the symmetry of color and structure. It has a typical pigment network (circle), regular dots and globules (arrows) but only one melanoma-specific criterion – a blue-white structure. The dots and globules at the periphery indicate an actively changing lesion. This is the type of pigmented skin lesion that needs clinical and dermoscopic follow-up.

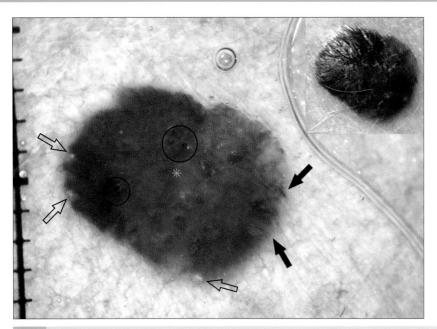

Figure 277 Seborrheic keratosis
Is there a blue-white structure (asterisk) here? Maybe there are some subtle streaks (solid arrows). There might be a few milia-like cysts (open arrows) and follicular openings (circles). So this lesion has melanoma-specific criteria and criteria seen in a seborrheic keratosis. Remember, if in doubt, cut it out.

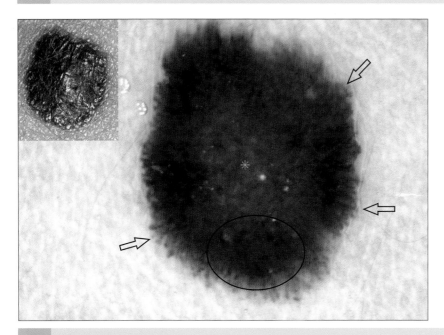

Figure 278 Spitz nevus
The differential diagnosis for this spitzoid appearance should include Spitz nevus and melanoma. There is a central blue-white structure (asterisk) and symmetrically oriented streaks (arrows) around the lesion. These features favor the diagnosis of a Spitz nevus. There are also irregular dots and globules (circle), which suggest a melanoma.

DARKER SKINNED RACES

GENERAL PRINCIPLES

- Dermoscopy criteria can be seen not only in skin phototype I–IV, but also in darker skinned races with skin phototypes V and VI.
- African–American, Haitian, Cuban, Indian, Central and South Americans are examples of darker skinned races in whom dermoscopy is a helpful technique.
- There is no reason why dermoscopy cannot be used on darker skinned races around the world.
- Congenital melanocytic nevi of any size, acquired melanocytic nevi, nail-apparatus pigmentation, acral pigmentation and vascular lesions benefit from dermoscopic evaluation in patients with skin phototype III–VI.
- Dermoscopy might not be helpful for heavily pigmented lesions.
- Global and local features should be evaluated carefully in all races.

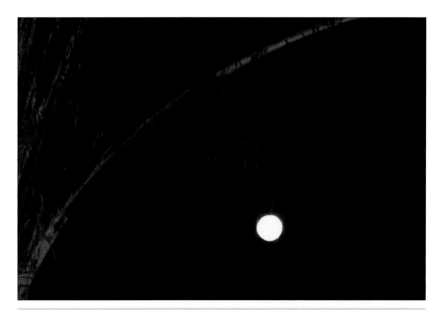

Moon over Miami, homogeneity at its finest. The ultimate homogeneous global pattern because it lacks the face of the man in the moon.

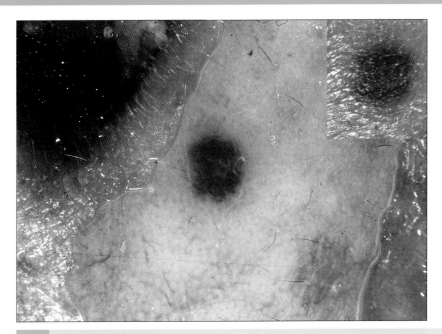

Figure 279 Blue nevus

This is a stereotypical blue nevus with a blue homogeneous global pattern in a 51-year-old Jamaican woman, skin phototype V. She has a family history of melanoma and was very worried about this lesion on her nose. After a confident dermoscopic diagnosis was made, the patient was reassured that she did not have melanoma and a scarring procedure in a cosmetically important area was avoided.

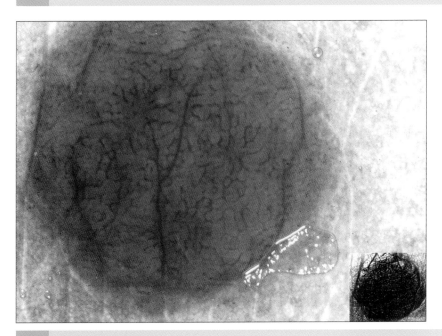

Figure 280 Nevus

There were no melanoma-specific criteria in this well circumscribed, banal appearing nevus on a Latino patient with skin phototype IV. It is a verrucous brown papule with pigmentation in the fissures of the skin. In all skin phototypes do not confuse pigmentation in skin fissures with an atypical pigment network.

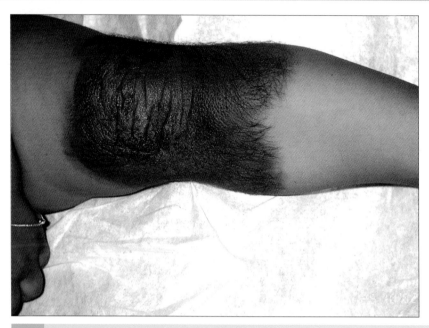

Figure 281 Congenital melanocytic nevus
This is a large congenital melanocytic nevus in a Latino teenager with skin phototype IV. Clinically it is not a thick lesion, so it is perfect for dermoscopic evaluation (see Figure 282).

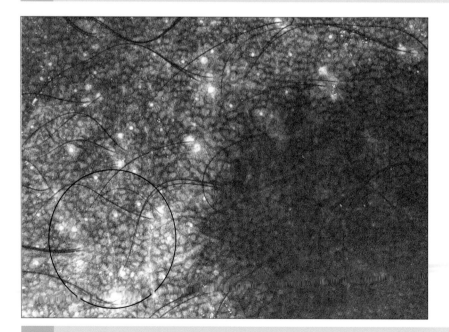

Figure 282 Congenital melanocytic nevus
Dermoscopic evaluation of the congenital melanocytic nevus shown in Figure 281 demonstrates several shades of brown and a typical pigment network (circle). It was possible to examine the entire lesion with dermoscopy. No melanoma-specific criteria were identified.

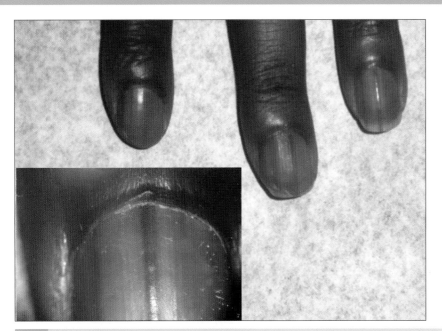

○
○
●
Figure 283 Banal nail-apparatus pigmentation
Dermoscopy is helpful for evaluating nail-apparatus pigmentation in all skin phototypes. In darker skinned races, nail-apparatus melanoma is more common. These clinical and dermoscopic images show pigmented bands in a Jamaican woman with skin phototype V. The proximal nailfold and pigmented band are more clearly seen with dermoscopy. In this case the history was important in diagnosing banal pigmented bands. The dermoscopic picture was completely benign, thus avoiding potentially disfiguring nail matrix biopsies.

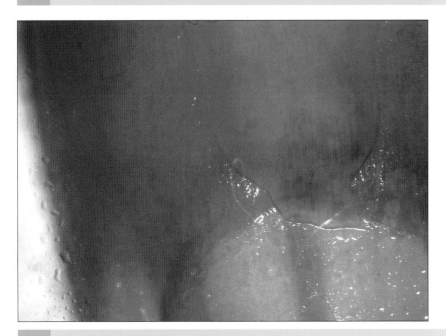

○
○
●
Figure 284 Banal nail-apparatus pigmentation
Here is the dermoscopic image of the proximal nailfold and proximal part of the pigmented band shown in Figure 283. No high-risk criteria such as multiple colors, irregular dots and globules or irregular band were seen.

BLUE LESIONS

GENERAL PRINCIPLES

- Blue color can be seen in benign and malignant lesions. They are not all blue nevi.
- Blue color indicates that melanin is deep in the dermis.
- It is imperative to develop a complete differential diagnosis for blue lesions.
- If you see a lesion with blue color but it also has other criteria, it should be evaluated like any other lesion.
- Blue lesions can be tricky. If in doubt, do not hesitate – cut it out.

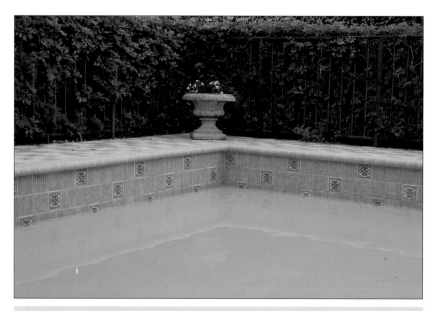

Blue-white structures can be fun, but not if they are in a pigmented skin lesion on your body.

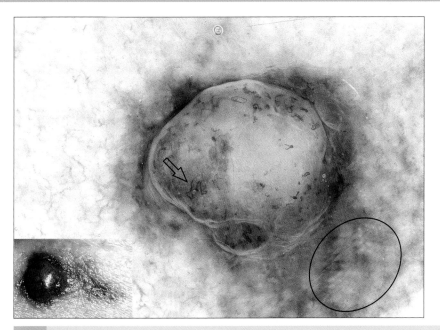

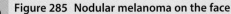

Figure 285 Nodular melanoma on the face

This lesion lacks criteria for a melanocytic lesion, seborrheic keratosis, basal cell carcinoma or hemangioma; therefore by definition it is melanocytic by exclusion. There may be some rhomboidal structures (circle) and the irregular linear vessels found in melanoma (arrow). The nodule has an obvious blue-white structure. This lesion has a high-risk dermoscopic picture and must be removed.

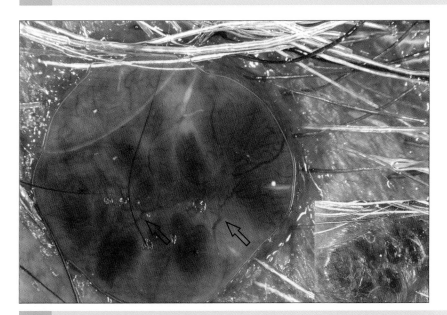

Figure 286 Basal cell carcinoma

This is a stereotypical basal cell carcinoma. There is an absence of criteria seen in melanocytic lesions and there are two criteria needed to diagnose a basal cell carcinoma – arborizing vessels (arrows) and blue-gray blotches (asterisks).

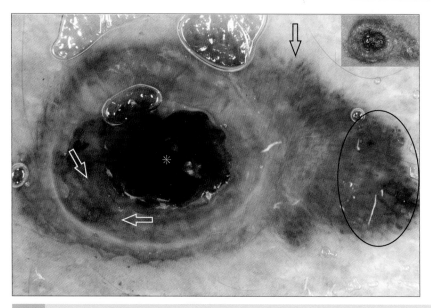

Figure 287 Melanoma

One's first impression might be that this is a basal cell carcinoma because of the ulceration (asterisk) and vessels (white arrows). Scan the lesion for all criteria. It actually has dots and globules (circle), so it is melanocytic. Now it is looking like a melanoma because of the blue-white structure, asymmetrically located irregular dots and globules, and irregular streaks (black arrow). This lesion therefore needs a histopathologic diagnosis. The dermoscopic picture will help in planning the surgical approach. It is important not to shave through this invasive melanoma.

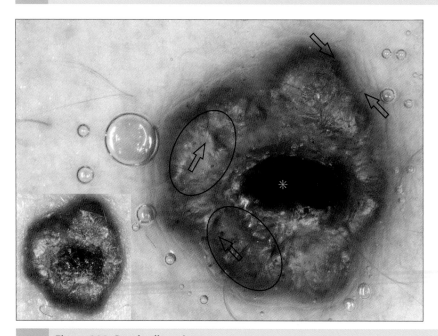

Figure 288 Basal cell carcinoma

This lesion is remarkably similar to that shown in Figure 287. Features include ulceration (asterisk), blue-white structures (circles) and a few irregular dots and globules (arrows). This lesion is melanocytic by definition if the rules are strictly followed, although it turned out to be a basal cell carcinoma. The important point is that this dermoscopic picture needs a histopathologic diagnosis.

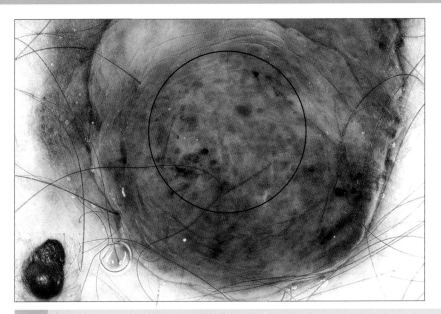

Figure 289 Melanoma
This lesion is similar to that shown in Figure 285. The melanoma-specific criteria are the extensive blue-white structure and irregular dots and globules (circle), of which most are purplish but a few are black. The color is not as important as the structure itself. Reddish dots and globules that are out of focus can be one of the vascular patterns seen in melanoma.

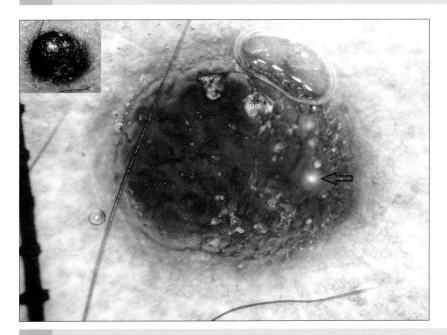

Figure 290 Blue nevus
This is a good example of a blue nevus with relatively homogeneous blue color. It is dry and scaly (asterisk) with milia-like cysts (arrow). Do not forget that the differential diagnosis includes nodular and cutaneous metastatic melanoma. The entire clinical picture will help one decide on the management of this lesion.

COMBINED NEVUS

GENERAL PRINCIPLES

- By definition a combined nevus is a blue nevus in conjunction with a more superficial regular melanocytic nevus.
- Various shades of blue and brown should raise suspicion of a combined nevus
- All 'fried egg'-appearing nevi, especially in children, are not high-risk lesions and dermoscopic examination can help prove this.

- A high-risk pigmented skin lesion can also have a 'fried egg' appearance so it is important always to look for high-risk dermoscopic criteria.
- There are many variations of the morphology seen with combined nevi. If in doubt, cut it out.

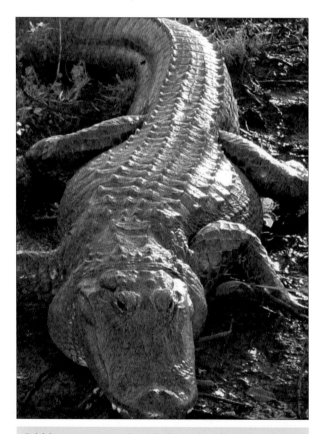

Cobblestone pattern Everglades style. Alligators demonstrate the angular structures that make up the benign cobblestone pattern. Yes, this alligator is alive but sleeping. Make the wrong move and things could become less benign because alligators can run as fast as a small dog. Focus your attention with this technique to protect your patients.

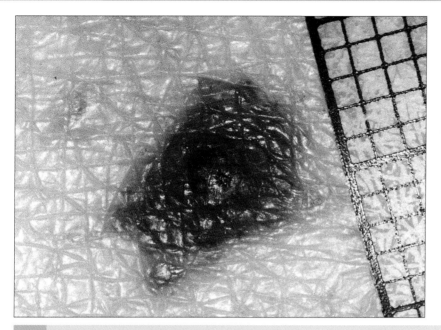

Figure 291 Combined nevus clinically suspicious for melanoma
This is a typical 'fried egg'-appearing nevus. The clinical history and dermoscopic appearance provide the best data for deciding on the lesion's management.

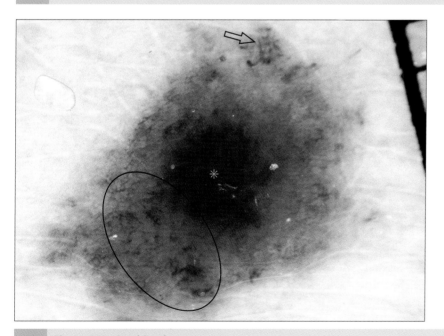

Figure 292 Combined nevus
This dermoscopic image of Figure 291 should be worrisome for the novice dermoscopist. There are three melanoma-specific criteria – a blue-white structure (asterisk), an atypical pigment network (circle) and irregular dots and globules (arrow). Although the criteria are subtle there are more than enough to warrant a histopathologic diagnosis. It is better to err on the side of caution and make a specific diagnosis with a dermoscopic picture like this.

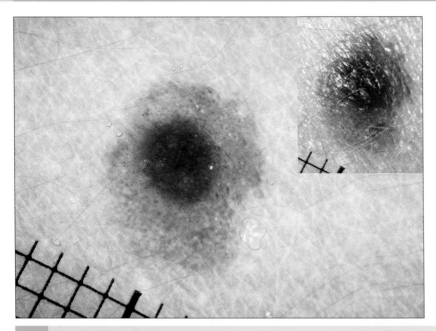

Figure 293 Combined nevus
This 'fried egg'-appearing nevus is less worrisome than the last case because the blue-white structure is symmetrical and well defined. The rest of the lesion is made up of small dots and globules – the globular global pattern.

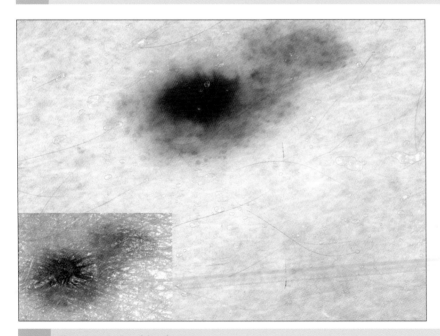

Figure 294 Combined nevus
Wherever there is asymmetry of color or structure, always raise one's index of suspicion that the lesion is high risk. The blue-white structure is asymmetrically located at the periphery. This is potentially a high-risk presentation. Consider asking for a second pathology opinion with this dermoscopic picture if the pathology report is low risk.

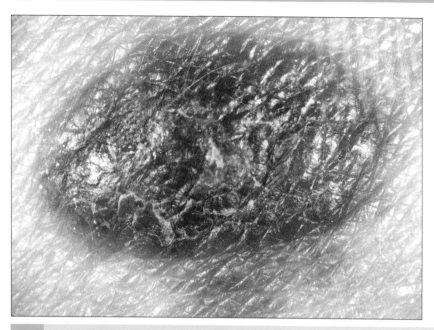

Figure 295 What is your diagnosis?

'Fried egg' nevus? 'Fried egg' melanoma? What should be done? Check it out with dermoscopy (see Figure 296).

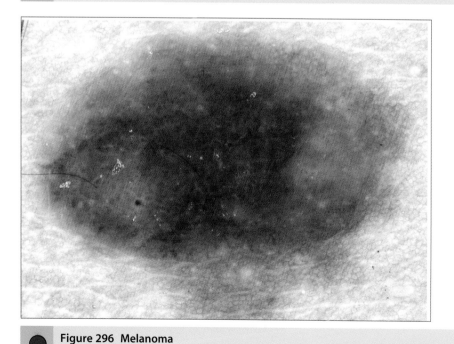

Figure 296 Melanoma

Find the melanoma-specific criteria in this lesion. The image demonstrates asymmetry of color and structure, a multicomponent global pattern, irregular dots and globules, and blue-white structures.

FLAT LESIONS ON THE FACE

GENERAL PRINCIPLES

- The clinical appearance and initial 'gut' impressions should not be ignored when evaluating flat brown lesions on the head and neck.
- Do not confuse the follicular ostia of a melanocytic lesion with the milia-like cysts of a seborrheic keratosis. Many times you will not be able to tell the difference.

- Do not expect to see 'classic' site-specific criteria. If there is a possible site-specific criterion, then consider it to be one.
- Many high-risk lesions on the head and neck area are relatively featureless. Look for subtle high-risk clues such as different shades of color asymmetrically located in the lesion.

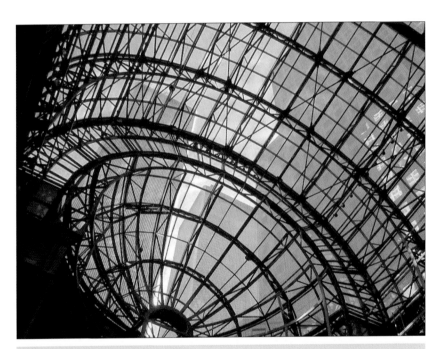

Steel network in the city, New York City.

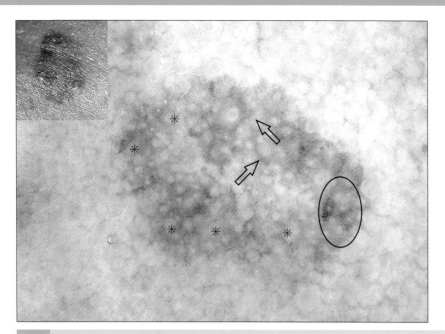

Figure 297 Lentigo maligna on the nose

Are the round-to-oval structures (asterisks) the milia-like cysts of a seborrheic keratosis or the follicular ostia of a melanocytic lesion? It is necessary to make this initial distinction. Are there any site-specific, melanoma-specific criteria? There are asymmetrically pigmented follicular openings (arrows) and no annular–granular structures. There are also early rhomboid structures (circle), but no gray network. The asymmetry of different shades of brown color is another important high-risk clue.

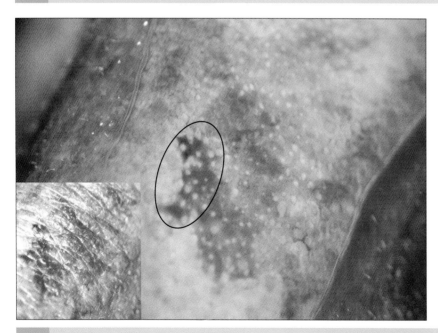

Figure 298 Solar lentigo on the nose

Once again one has to decide what the round yellow structures are. Is this a melanocytic or non-melanocytic lesion? There are no site-specific, melanoma-specific criteria. There is, however, asymmetry of different shades of brown color. The concavity of the border's 'moth-eaten' appearance (circle) is a clue to the correct diagnosis. The clinical appearance together with the asymmetry of color are enough to warrant a histopathologic diagnosis. Some high-risk lesions on the head and neck can be relatively featureless.

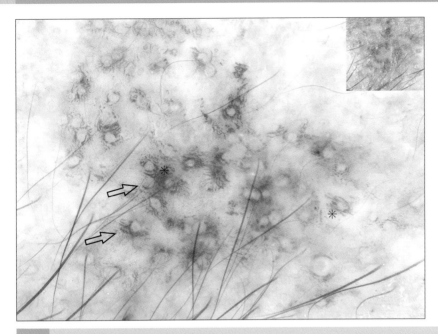

Figure 299 Flat seborrheic keratosis
This image shows asymmetry of color and structure with two site-specific, melanoma-specific criteria – asymmetrically pigmented follicular openings (arrows) and annular–granular structures (asterisks). In this case these were false-positive high-risk criteria. A second opinion on the pathology should be considered with this benign lesion.

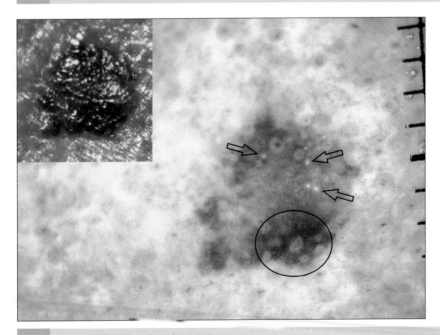

Figure 300 Seborrheic keratosis
Although this shows asymmetry of color and structure and a suggestion of rhomboid structures (circle), the definite, stereotypical milia-like cysts (arrows) allow the diagnosis. Remember, milia-like cysts can be seen in melanocytic lesions. If in doubt, cut it out.

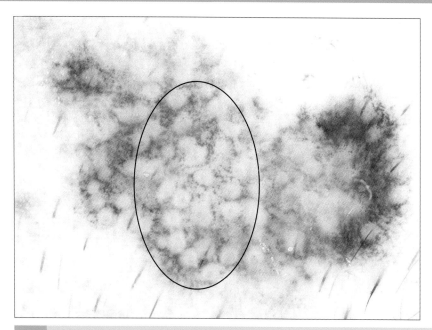

Figure 301 Lichen planus-like keratosis

It is necessary to develop a differential diagnosis for all dermoscopic criteria and such knowledge is needed for difficult-to-diagnose lesions like this. There are multiple bluish dots and globules (circle). They are annular–granular structures made up of melanophages. Melanophages can be seen in melanocytic, non-melanocytic benign or malignant lesions. The extensiveness of the melanophages points to a benign lesion.

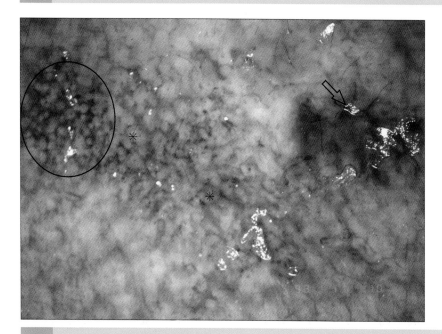

Figure 302 Lentigo maligna

This lesion shows annular–granular structures (asterisks), asymmetrically pigmented follicles, rhomboid structures (circle) and an asymmetrically located blue-white structure (arrow). In summary, it is a stereotypical lentigo maligna. Many not-so-obvious, flat, high-risk lesions are seen on the face; therefore have a high index of suspicion for any pigmented macule or patch on the head or neck of older patients.

NODULAR LESIONS ON THE FACE

GENERAL PRINCIPLES

- The differential diagnosis of pigmented and non-pigmented nodules on the face includes melanocytic, non-melanocytic, benign and malignant lesions. Quite often, the clinical appearance is non-specific, and dermoscopy will help in making a clinical diagnosis.
- Nodules often have ridges and fissures. Do not confuse pigmentation in the fissures with an atypical pigment network.
- A macular component to a nodular lesion should raise the index of suspicion that the lesion could be high risk.

- A soft compressible nodule that can be easily moved from side to side favors low-risk pathology. Do not hesitate to palpate or squash lesions down and move them from side with the instrumentation used.
- The main differential diagnosis for nodular lesions on the face are nevi and basal cell carcinomas. Nodular melanoma is rarely found in this area.

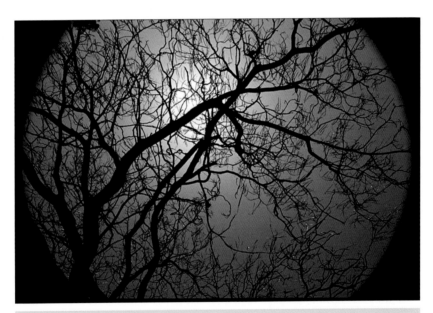

The vessels characteristic of a basal cell carcinoma are described as 'arborizing' because they look exactly like this.

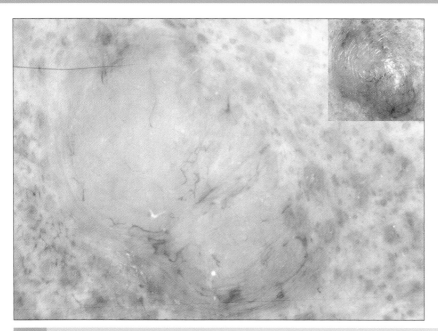

Figure 303 Basal cell carcinoma

A pigment network, dots and globules and streaks are not seen, so consider this to be a non-melanocytic lesion. Some nevi can have this dermoscopic picture, but are usually soft and can be easily moved from side to side. Clinically this looks like a basal cell carcinoma. There are some larger vessels, but they are not the stereotypical arborizing ones. Rarely amelanotic melanoma looks like this.

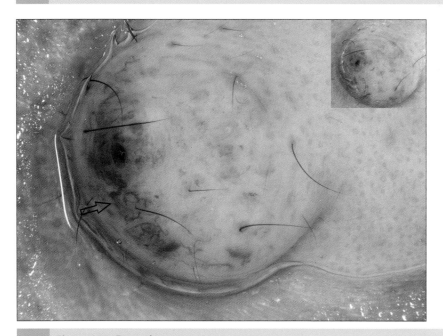

Figure 304 Dermal nevus

Pink color – beware. Soft, movable lesion – relax. Although there are definite arborizing vessels (arrow), the history and soft nodule point to benign pathology. If in doubt, cut it out. By the way, hairs are never seen in a basal cell carcinoma.

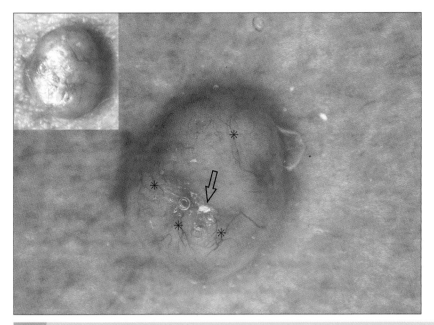

Figure 305 Basal cell carcinoma

What criteria are seen here? A milia-like cyst (arrow) or a scale? There are also arborizing vessels (asterisks) and an asymmetrical border of pigmentation. These are confusing criteria, so it is best to find out what the lesion is more specifically.

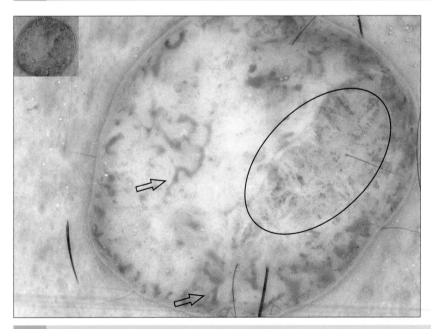

Figure 306 Dermal nevus

This lesion has globules (circle) and arborizing vessels (arrows) – criteria for a melanocytic lesion and a basal cell carcinoma. What is the history? If the patient is a young adult, a nevus is more likely, but if this is on an adult seriously consider basal cell carcinoma. Hairs are never seen in a basal cell carcinoma.

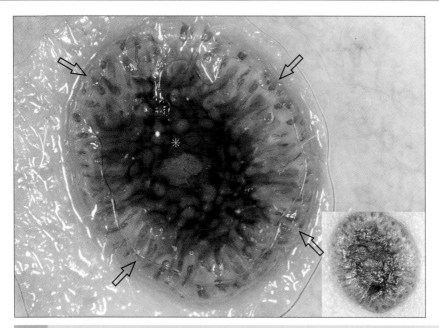

Figure 307 Keratoacanthoma

This lesion has a spitzoid or starburst global appearance, with white blue-white structures and vessels at the periphery (arrows) and central branched (asterisk) and thickened hyperpigmentation. Symmetry like this is not seen in melanomas and the vessels are not the dotted or irregular linear ones also found in melanoma. Rarely a rapidly growing nodule turns out to be an aggressive melanoma. In this case it was a keratoacanthoma.

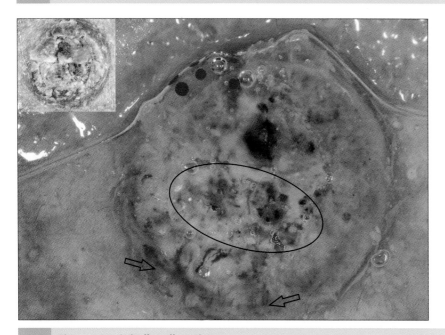

Figure 308 Spindle cell carcinoma

This lesion looks very worrisome. Overall there is asymmetry of color and structure, and both white and pink color can be seen, so increasing the index of suspicion that this is a high-risk lesion even further. In addition there is an irregular blotch and there are irregular dots and globules (circle) plus a high-risk dotted and linear (arrows) vascular pattern. This needs to be excised as soon as possible.

FEATURELESS MELANOMA

GENERAL PRINCIPLES
- There can be high-risk lesions without obvious high-risk criteria.
- Completely featureless lesions are rarely found.
- Know the entire history.
- Does the lesion look high risk clinically?
- Is it an 'ugly duckling' lesion or are there other similar-appearing lesions? Increase the index of suspicion if it is the 'ugly duckling' and differs from other lesions.
- Develop a differential diagnosis for all global and local patterns and criteria.
- Think things through.
- Ask a colleague for his or her opinion. Two minds are often better than one.
- Is there subtle asymmetry of color and structure?
- Do the colors or structures appear smudged or out of focus? If so this could mean it is a high-risk lesion.
- White color – beware.
- Pink color – beware.
- Look for melanoma-specific vascular patterns.
- The patient's luck and your high index of suspicion can be life-saving.

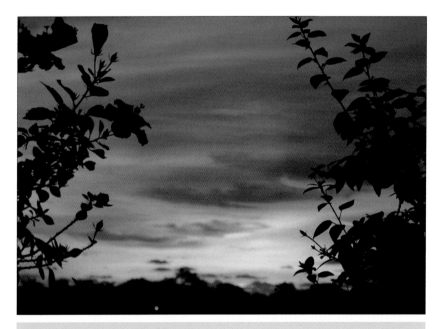

Beautiful, isn't it? Pink color beware!

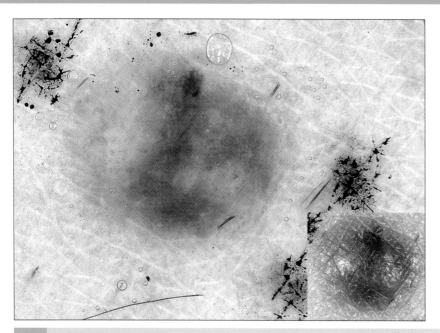

Figure 309 Melanoma

By default, this is a melanocytic lesion because it lacks criteria for any other lesion such as a basal cell carcinoma or seborrheic keratosis. The colors are smudged or out of focus. There is also asymmetry of color and structure. White color – beware.

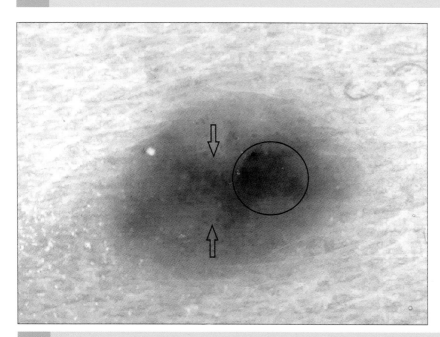

Figure 310 Melanoma

Pink color – beware. The small reddish dots (arrows) could be one of the vascular patterns seen in melanoma. Is the grayish blotch (circle) created by macrophages in the papillary dermis or pigmented melanoma cells? (Figure courtesy of MA Pizzichetta, Aviano, Italy.)

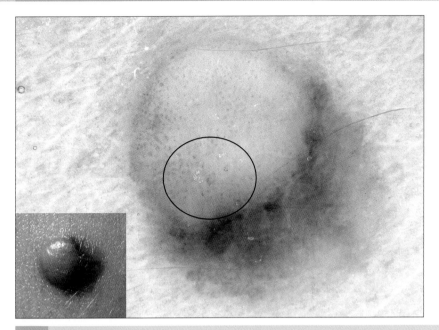

Figure 311 Melanoma
This is a melanocytic lesion because there is an absence of obvious criteria to diagnose other lesions. White color – beware. Do not mistake it for the central white patch of a dermatofibroma. There is also pink color and the small dotted (circle) melanoma-specific vascular pattern. All of these subtle criteria spell melanoma until proven otherwise.

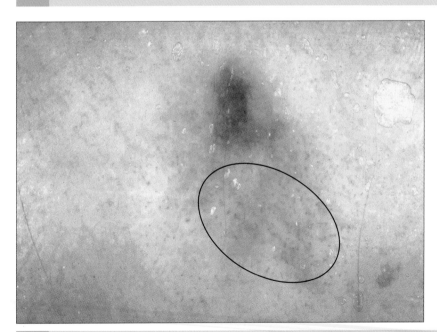

Figure 312 Melanoma
This is a subtle and difficult case. Could this be a collision lesion? Pink color – beware. Is this an 'ugly duckling' lesion? Look to see if the patient has other similar lesions. It is less worrisome if so. The small red dots of the melanoma-specific vascular pattern (circle) can be seen. Is the color gray or brown, and does it matter? Gray could represent the melanophages seen in regressing melanomas. The colors in this lesion plus the dotted vascular pattern are sufficient clues to warrant a histologic diagnosis. (Figure courtesy of MA Pizzichetta, Aviano, Italy.)

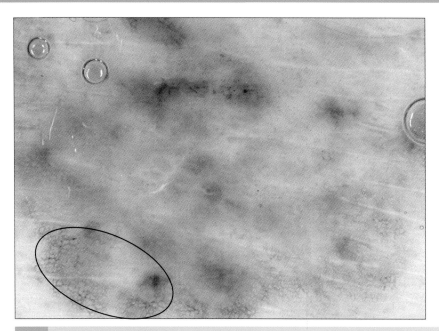

Figure 313 Melanoma

A pigment network (circle) is seen, so by definition this is a melanocytic lesion. There is white color, but it is the same intensity as in the surrounding skin. It does not fit the definition of a blue-white structure, which should be whiter than the surrounding skin. There is subtle pink color and a broken up branched network (circle). All of the colors and the structure are smudged and out of focus when this is looked at closely and there is significant asymmetry of color and structure.

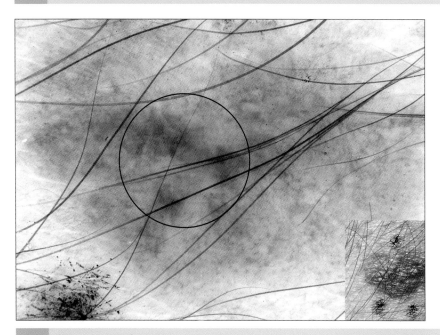

Figure 314 Melanoma

The only clues here that this might be a high-risk lesion are the gray blotches (circle), which could be melanophages in a regressing melanoma, and the suggestion of white color. A high index of suspicion and these clues should lead to an excision.

FOLLOW-UP OF MELANOCYTIC LESIONS

GENERAL PRINCIPLES

- Create a database of lesions to follow over time.
- Most high-risk patients should be seen every 6 months to look for dermoscopic changes over time.
- Most lesions do not change over time.
- Changes are not always an indication for excision.

- There are no data on the significant changes over time in pediatric or pregnant patients. Treat them as you would treat other patients.
- Significant changes over time include development of an asymmetrical enlargement, the appearance of melanoma-specific criteria, new colors and the disappearance of criteria.

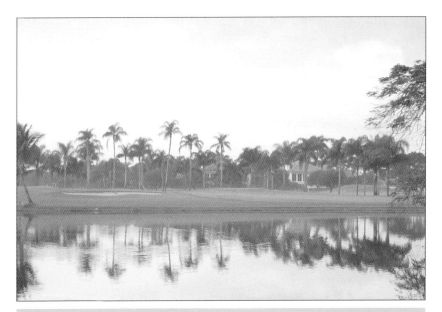

A side-by-side comparison can be good or bad. In this case it is 'quite' good.

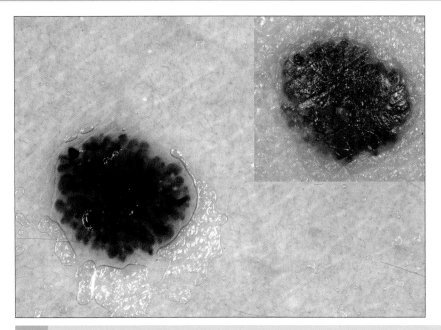

○
○
○
Figure 315 Spitz nevus
This is a classic starburst pattern of a Spitz nevus in a young patient with a symmetrical rim of dots and globules plus streaks at all points along the periphery of the lesion.

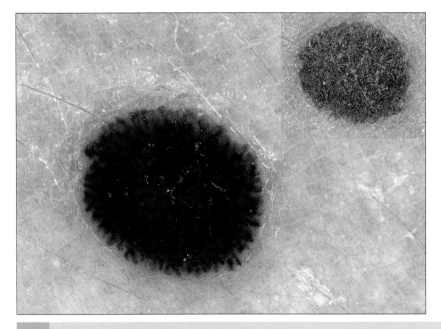

○
○
○
Figure 316 Spitz nevus
Note the change in the lesion shown in Figure 315 over 9 months. Such changes are rarely seen unless Spitz nevi are monitored and not excised. Clearly the lesion has enlarged symmetrically and the rim of streaks is much smaller and more distinct.

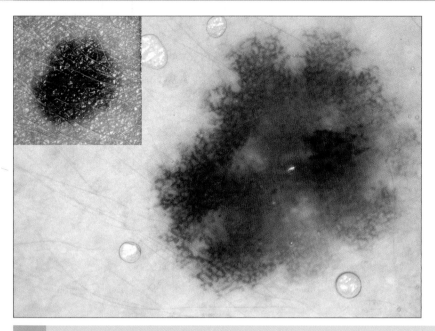

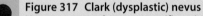

Figure 317 Clark (dysplastic) nevus
How many melanoma-specific criteria are there here? It is unusual not to excise a lesion with so much asymmetry of color and structure.

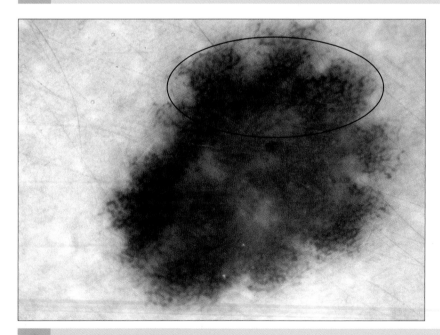

Figure 318 Clark (dysplastic) nevus
At follow-up of the lesion shown in Figure 317, it can be seen that the lesion is larger and has a darker color with a more prominent pigment network (circle). The irregular blotch that had dots and globules in it is no longer present. The significant changes illustrated in these two images warrant excision of the lesion.

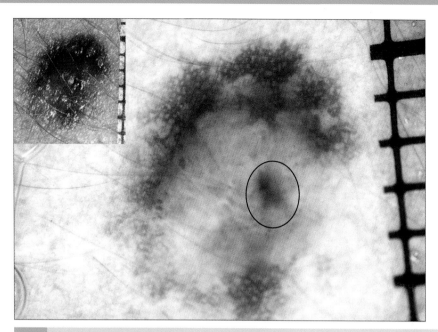

Figure 319 Combined nevus

The white color, asymmetry of color and structure, and atypical pigment network of this lesion are all high-risk criteria. Is that a blotch (circle) or part of a blue-white structure? Are you surprised that we did not excise this lesion?

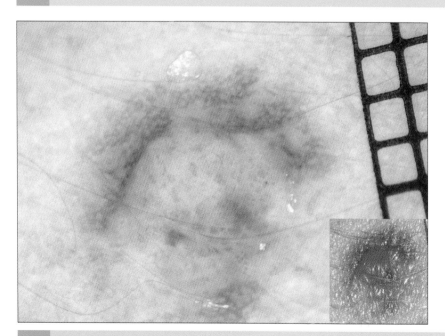

Figure 320 Combined nevus

This is a follow-up image of the lesion shown in Figure 319. Is everything actually looking better over time or is this a regressing melanoma? Clinically there is a soft, compressible, skin-colored nodule present, so the white color is not a sign of regression. Would you excise this lesion now or continue to follow it over time?

INKSPOT LENTIGO

GENERAL PRINCIPLES

- Clinically and dermoscopically inkspot lentigines have a very characteristic appearance.
- Typically an inkspot lentigo is black and sharply demarcated with a bizarre-looking pigment network filling the lesion. There is an absence of other criteria.
- Individuals with inkspot lentigines commonly have fair skin, light hair and light eyes, and are at risk of developing melanoma. Don't forget to do a comprehensive skin examination to look for high-risk pigmented skin lesions.
- Inkspot lentigines are usually located on the upper trunk and extremities and are surrounded by regular or large sunburn freckles.
- On seeing an 'inkspot lentigo' try not to miss seeing the presence of any melanoma-specific criteria.
- If in doubt, cut it out.

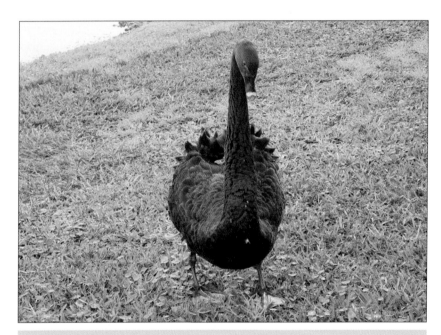

An angry black spot.

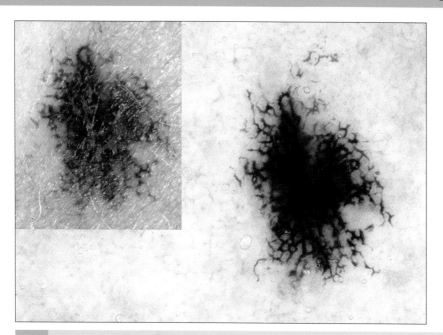

Figure 321 Inkspot lentigo

This is a variation of the morphology seen in an inkspot lentigo characterized by a bizarre pigment network. There is also a large homogeneous area with a gray color representing melanophages in the papillary dermis.

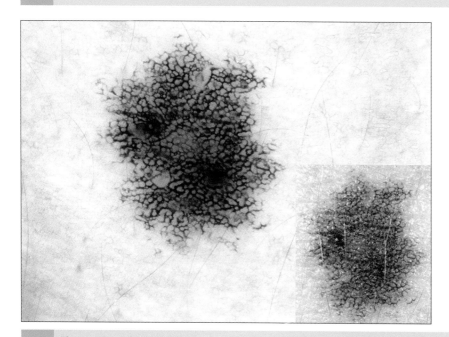

Figure 322 Inkspot lentigo

This is a stereotypical inkspot lentigo. The network is commonly black.

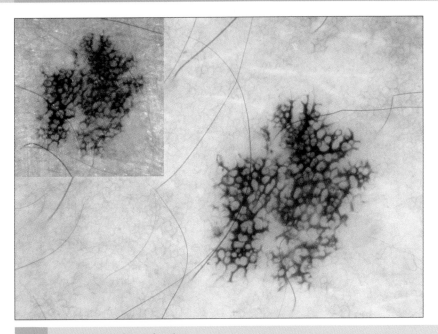

Figure 323 Inkspot lentigo
A third variation of the appearance of inkspot lentigo. The clinical appearance, dark color, bizarre shape of the pigment network and absence of other criteria suggest the correct diagnosis.

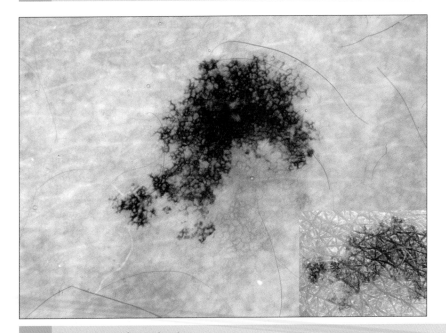

Figure 324 Inkspot lentigo
This picture is worrisome because of the asymmetry of color and structure, the irregular dots and globules and the irregular blotch. It is not wrong to biopsy a lesion that looks like this.

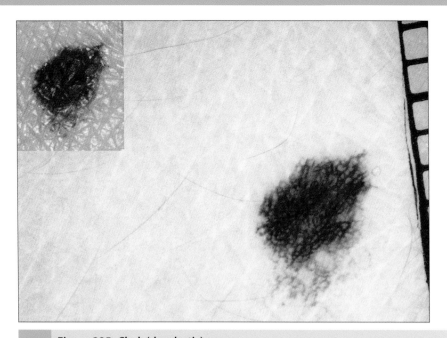

Figure 325 Clark (dysplastic) nevus
The quality of the pigment network is suggestive of a reticular type of Clark (dysplastic) nevus. The pigment network is atypical and the color is blotchy.

Therefore, excision or digital follow-up is recommended.

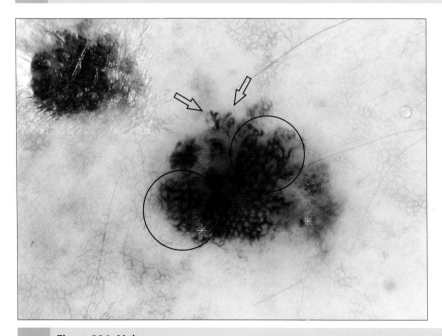

Figure 326 Melanoma
This lesion is black with a pigment network, but these are the only features this melanoma has in common with an inkspot lentigo. This lesion has prominent melanoma-specific criteria – an atypical pigment network (circles), irregular dots and globules (asterisks) and subtle streaks (arrows).

MUCOSAL LESIONS

GENERAL PRINCIPLES

- Most pigmented lesions on mucosal surfaces are low risk.
- Determine whether the lesion is black, brown, blue or red.
- Red–blue color – non-melanocytic.
- Brown–black color – melanocytic.

- If a pigmented skin lesion looks worrisome clinically, shows asymmetry of color and structure and has melanoma-specific criteria it does not matter where on the body it is located. These criteria are high risk and warrant a histopathologic diagnosis.

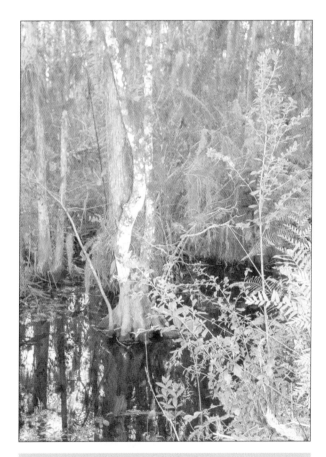

There are streaks, asymmetry and dull color. What you can't see are the alligators hidden below the surface. Don't miss important criteria!

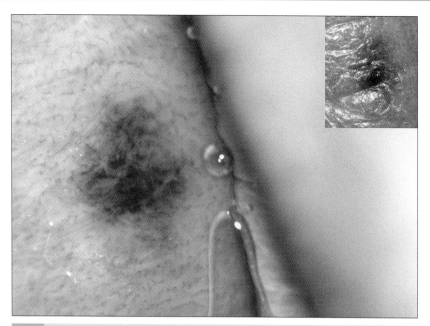

Figure 327 Labial lentigo
This mucosal lesion shows asymmetry of color and structure, irregular dots and globules, and an irregular blotch of pigmentation. Overall this is a worrisome dermoscopic picture for the lip and warrants histopathologic diagnosis.

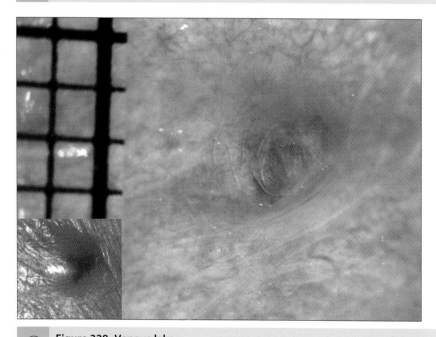

Figure 328 Venous lake
This is a stereotypical venous lake with a homogeneous dark-blue color. The patient can be reassured that this is benign once it has been squashed down easily and the color disappears.

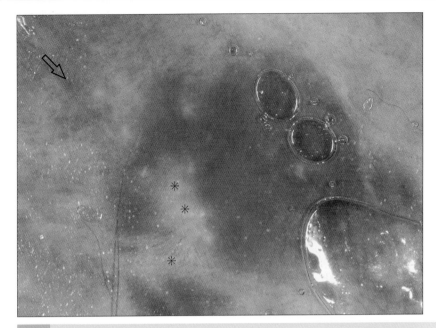

Figure 329 Lentigo
This is a very worrisome dermoscopic picture because of the blue-white structure (asterisks), remnants of parallel pigment pattern (arrow) and multiple shades of color. Fortunately this was not a melanoma. Make sure a good dermatopathologist analyses the histologic specimen for this dermoscopic picture.

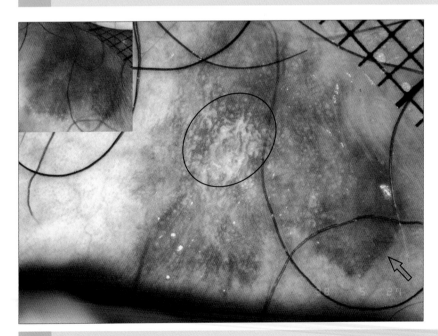

Figure 330 Labial lentigo
Here is another worrisome dermoscopic picture because of the asymmetry of color and structure, the atypical pigment network (circle), the scar-like central area and the irregular blotch (arrow) asymmetrically located at the border.

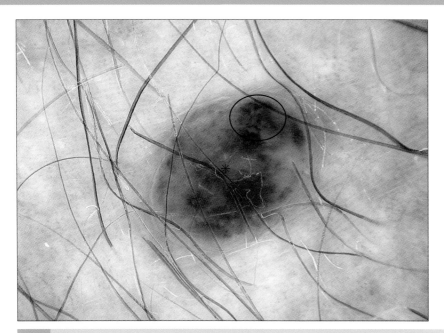

Figure 331 Genital nevus

This small papule on the vulva shows irregular blotches and a pink color. Irregular blotches plus pink color indicate the need for excision. In one area (circle) there is a subtle pigment network indicating that this is a melanocytic lesion. A blue-white structure is also seen (asterisk). The differential diagnosis includes melanoma or Clark (dysplastic) nevus, so this lesion should be excised.

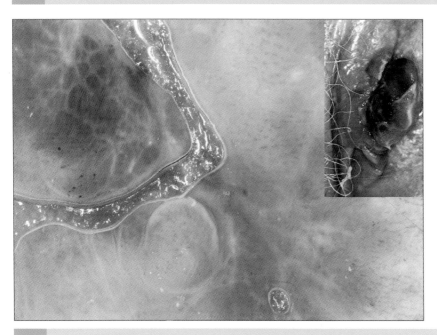

Figure 332 Melanoma

This is a melanoma of the vulva. No other diagnosis should come to mind on seeing this clinical and dermoscopic picture. This large asymmetrical lesion shows blue-white structures and irregular dots and globules.

MULTIPLE CLARK (DYSPLASTIC) NEVI

GENERAL PRINCIPLES

- Examining multiple nevi with dermoscopy is cost-effective and provides information about whether a patient has multiple high-risk or banal nevi.
- Most patients with multiple nevi have low-risk lesions, but this can be confirmed by checking them out with dermoscopy.
- Ask patients whether they have any new or changing nevi. Never ignore the patient's history.

- The 'ugly duckling' pigmented skin lesion seen both clinically and with dermoscopy warrants a histopathologic diagnosis.
- If a patient has multiple high-risk-looking lesions with dermoscopy, excise one or two to make a dermoscopic–pathologic correlation.
- The true number of melanomas is small compared to the number of patients with multiple dysplastic nevi. The vast majority do not need to be excised, but can be followed using digital systems to look for significant changes over time.

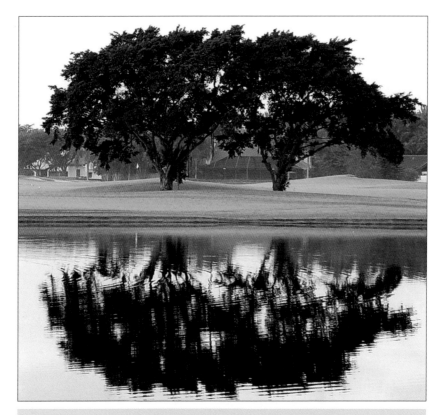

Keep this beautiful scene in your mind when trying to determine the symmetry or asymmetry of color and structure in a lesion. Is one side of a lesion the mirror image of the other?

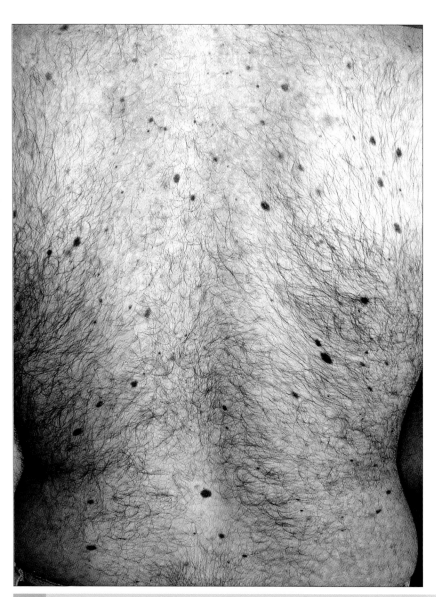

Figure 333 Multiple nevi
This is a stereotypical example of a person with multiple nevi. Clinically they look low risk, but he could have a melanoma. It is possible to examine most of these lesions rapidly with dermoscopy and obtain clues to point to high-risk lesions that do not look high risk clinically. These are usually the early melanomas that offer patients their best chances of survival. Dermoscopy opens up a new world of colors and structures that help in managing this common, difficult and serious problem (see Figures 334–337).

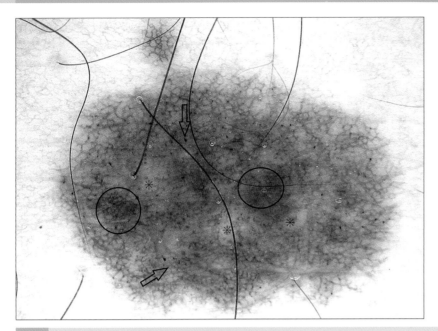

Figure 334 Clark (dysplastic) nevus
Here is an example of dysplastic nevus from the individual shown in Figure 333. Multifocal hypo-pigmentation (asterisks), atypical pigment network (circles) and irregular dots and globules (arrows) are seen. In the realm of dysplastic nevi, dermoscopic findings do not always correlate with pathology. Very worrisome lesions often turn out to be mildly dysplastic, whereas relatively featureless lesions may be revealed histopathologically to be severely dysplastic.

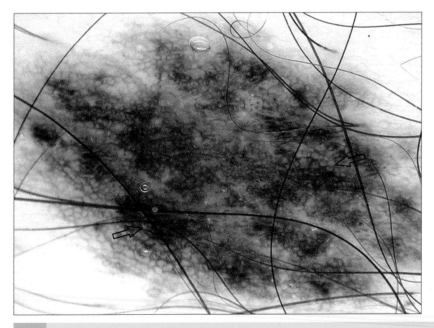

Figure 335 Clark (dysplastic) nevus
A similar pattern of dermoscopic criteria to those observed in Figure 334 can be seen in this nevus. The irregular blotches (arrows) point to a potentially more high-risk dysplastic nevus. Excision or digital follow-up examination are two ways to manage this lesion.

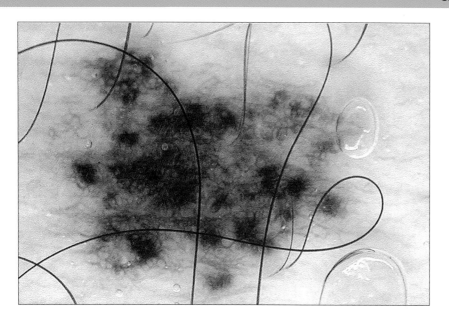

Figure 336 Clark (dysplastic) nevus

An 'ugly duckling' lesion that stands out has still not been found in this patient, who appears to have relatively similar-looking nevi. Which one should be excised to make a dermoscopic–pathologic correlation?

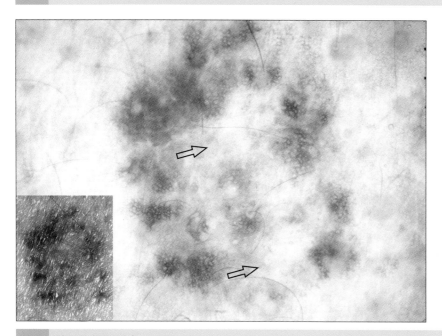

Figure 337 Melanoma

Here is the 'ugly ducking', however. This reddish, relatively featureless lesion differs from the others the man has. Note the multifocal hypopigmentation (arrows) verging on regression areas and atypical pigment network. Excision is mandatory. This high-risk lesion with dermoscopy can easily be overlooked if the patient is examined with the naked eye or using the typical magnification clinicians use. Melanomas will be missed less often if dermoscopy is mastered.

PIGMENTED LESIONS OF THE NAILS

GENERAL PRINCIPLES

- Dermoscopy makes the nail apparatus clearer.
- Nail-apparatus melanoma (NAM) accounts for 1–2% of melanomas in the lighter skinned population and 15–20% of melanomas in darker skinned races.
- Amelanotic NAM exists, so pink color – beware.
- High-risk dermoscopic criteria suggestive of NAM include asymmetry of color and structure, irregular pigmented bands, irregular blotches, irregular dots and globules, and Hutchinson's sign.
- Blood can be found in NAM, so look for high-risk criteria if you find blood in the nail.
- The chance of finding high-risk pathology in the pediatric population is low; therefore a worrisome history might be more important than a high-risk dermoscopic appearance.

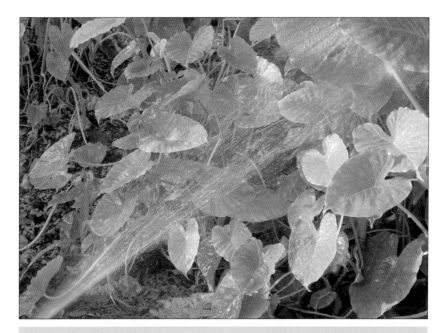

Uniform bands are good. Irregular bands can be bad.

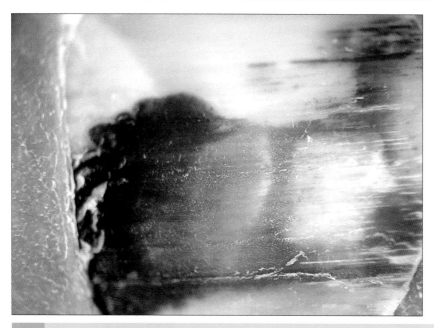

Figure 338 Hemorrhage

The purple diffuse blotch shown here is the color of dried blood. The linear areas and dots are worrisome – more so if they are brown. Hopefully, the history will point to some form of trauma to the nail. Follow the patient to ensure that the color grows distally with a normal nail proximally.

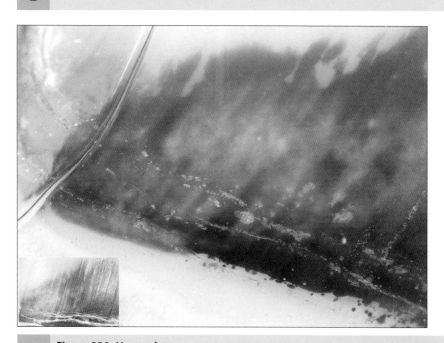

Figure 339 Hemorrhage

This image shows another variation of the morphology seen with blood. The purple color is important. It is well demarcated and relatively structureless. Hemorrhage can present as diffuse blotches, dots and globules, and streaks. The whitish color represents the hyperkeratosis seen in the nail plate. White color can be seen with scarring or hyperkeratosis. It is not always an ominous dermoscopic criterion.

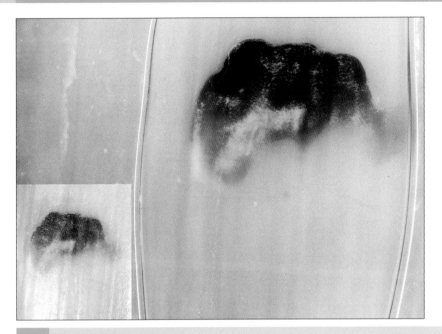

Figure 340 Hemorrhage
The dark dried blood in this nail is well demarcated, featureless and in the middle of the nail plate. It is growing out. Follow patients carefully to avoid missing NAM masquerading as blood.

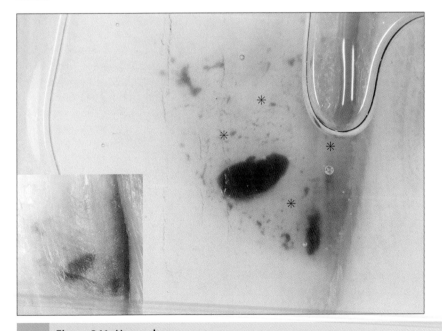

Figure 341 Hemorrhage
There are many faces of nail-apparatus hemorrhage. Always look for high-risk criteria before diagnosing pure hemorrhage. Here the reddish blotches of blood are in a jelly-like area of decomposing blood (asterisks).

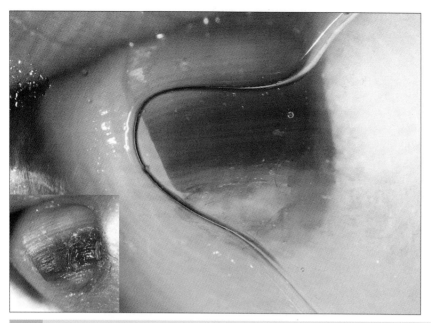

Figure 342 Nevus

The history of this lesion, age and race of the patient should be considered together with the dermoscopic picture before deciding on the management of nail-apparatus pigmentation. In this case there is uniform color and uniform linearity of the bands – a benign feature in most cases.

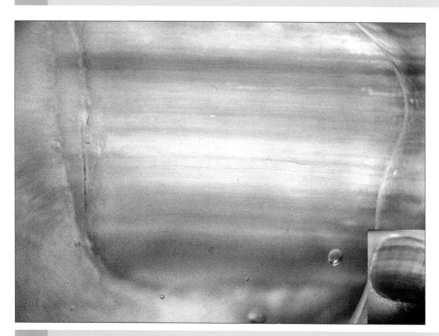

Figure 343 Melanoma

In a young patient, this irregularly pigmented band has not been correlated with high-risk pathology. In an adult, a solitary pigmented band with different shades of brown and different widths of the lines is high risk and requires a histopathologic diagnosis.

This is a stereotypical example of a high-risk nail-apparatus dermoscopic picture. It is necessary to focus attention to find these significant changes. Note the pigmentation on the skin – a positive Hutchinson's sign.

LESIONS WITH REGRESSION

GENERAL PRINCIPLES

- A bone-white color often represents scarring seen in regression.
- Do not confuse hypopigmentation with regression.
- A blue-white veil is a bluish groundglass-appearing area that can also be seen with regression.
- At times it is not possible to tell whether one is dealing with a white area of regression or a blue-white veil. These can now be diagnosed as blue-white structures.
- Blue-white structures are high-risk criteria seen in melanomas or Spitz nevi.
- Superficial spreading melanomas often have areas of regression.
- If even a hint of a blue-white structure is identified, it is better to err on the side of caution and make a histopathologic diagnosis.

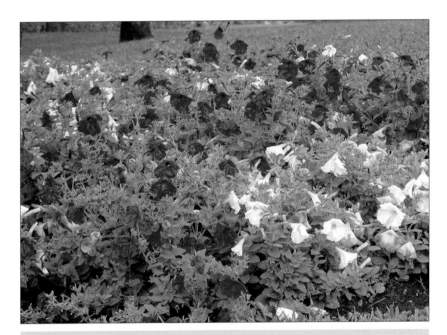

Blue-white structures.

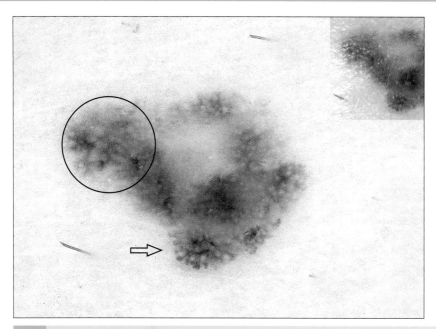

Figure 344 Melanoma

The white color is similar to the surrounding skin; therefore by definition it is not a regression area, which should be lighter than the surrounding skin. There is asymmetry of color and structure, atypical pigment network (circle) and a focus of streaks (arrow). Overall these criteria mean that the lesion should be excised. It is common for the novice dermoscopist to overdiagnose regression areas.

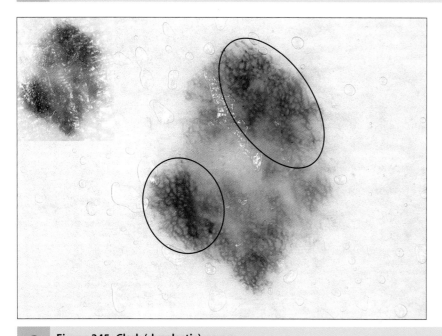

Figure 345 Clark (dysplastic) nevus

This case is similar to that shown in Figure 344. The light color is not light enough to be considered a regression area. The pigment network is atypical (circles). Multifocal hypopigmentation is commonly found in dysplastic nevi. This is the classic dermoscopic picture of a dysplastic nevus.

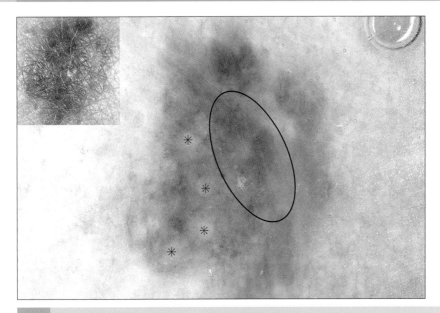

Figure 346 Melanoma

Pink color – beware. Asymmetry of color and structure – beware. The blue-white structure, which is whitish in this case within the pink zone, is an area of regression (circle). The oval white areas may or may not be areas of regression or hypopigmentation (asterisks). Pink with white color is high risk and by itself warrants a histologic diagnosis.

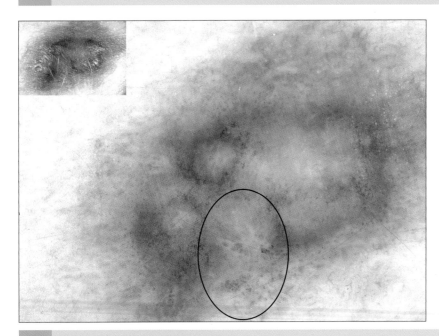

Figure 347 Clark (dysplastic) nevus

Pink color is high risk, but not 100% diagnostic of melanoma. The white color is not true scarring because it is the color of the surrounding skin. There are small reddish dots and globules in a pink zone (circle). This is a milky-red area – a high-risk vascular pattern. A second pathologic opinion was requested when this was first diagnosed as a benign nevus. Always try to make a good dermoscopic–pathologic correlation. If there is divergence, get a second pathologic opinion.

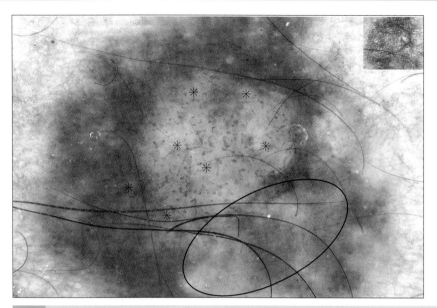

Figure 348 Melanoma

This melanoma has a stereotypical blue-white structure (asterisks). Melanophages, which are often found in regressing melanomas, are also seen in a whitish area (circle). As there is also asymmetry of color and structure, this should be considered to be a melanoma until proven otherwise.

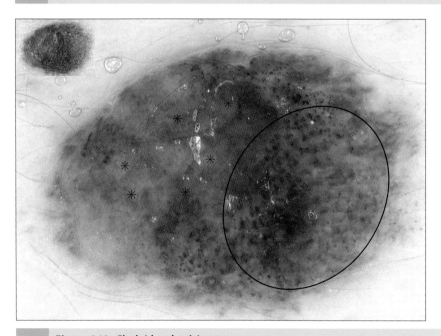

Figure 349 Clark (dysplastic) nevus

Here is another good example of a blue-white structure (asterisks). There are also remnants of a globular pattern with a large area of uniform dots and globules (circle). The dermoscopic–pathologic correlation of a benign lesion is not good. High-risk criteria are not always found in high-risk lesions. Do not be discouraged if an apparently high-risk lesion turns out not to be high risk.

RETICULAR LESIONS

GENERAL PRINCIPLES

- Take a bird's eye (global) view of the entire lesion to get a first impression.
- Reticular pattern = significant areas with pigment network.
- Is the pigment network typical or atypical?
- What other criteria are there to make the dermoscopic diagnosis?

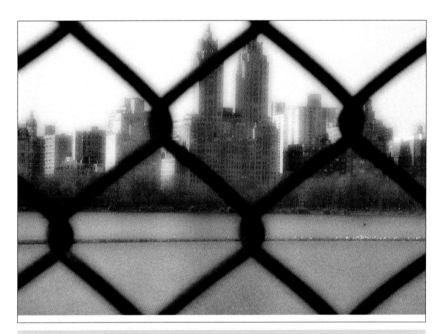

A pigment network fence, ground glass lake and skyscraper streaks in the city, New York City.

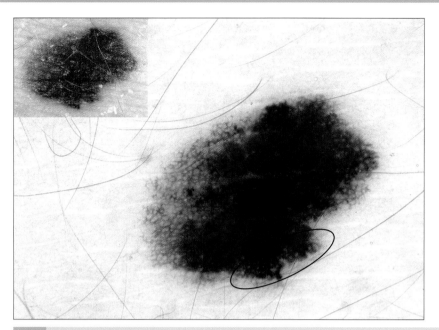

Figure 350 Melanoma

Surprisingly this turned out to be an in-situ melanoma. It does not look that worrisome. There is enough pigment network to say it has a reticular pattern, and the pigment network is slightly atypical. The subtle irregular streaks (circle) push this lesion over the edge to be malignant. Statistically a lesion with this dermoscopic picture would not be a melanoma, but a Clark (dysplastic) nevus. It is suspicious enough to warrant a histopathologic diagnosis.

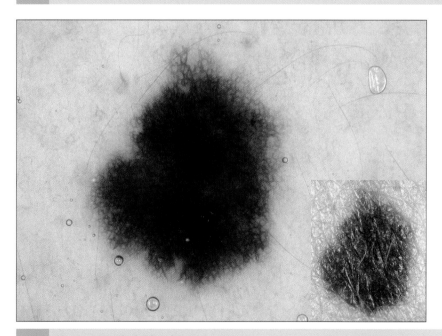

Figure 351 Clark (dysplastic) nevus

The pigment network fills most of this lesion. It has more of a reticular pattern than that shown in Figure 350. The pigment network and dots and globules are questionably atypical, but not strikingly worrisome. Differentiate this benign nevus from the in-situ melanoma in Figure 350. Here the network lines are thin and fade out at the periphery, in contrast to the previous case.

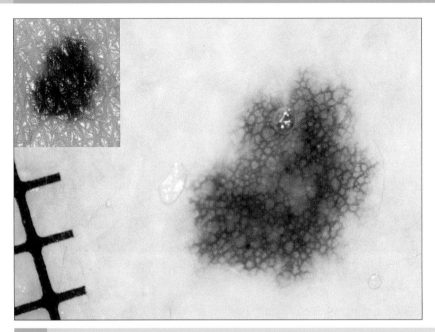

Figure 352 Clark (dysplastic) nevus

The pigment network is slightly atypical in this lesion because the line segments are thicker, branched and broken up. There are no other melanoma-specific criteria. Do not confuse the central area of hypopigmentation with a blue-white structure. Statistically, this picture is seen most often with Clark (mildly dysplastic) nevi.

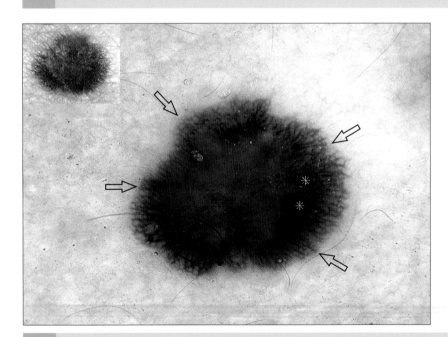

Figure 353 Spitz nevus

This lesion looks more ominous with a reticular pattern forming a starburst pattern. There are streaks at all border points along the periphery (arrows). This favors the diagnosis of a Spitz nevus. Blue-white structures can be seen in both Spitz nevi and melanomas. Melanoma-specific criteria include irregular dots and globules (asterisks) and irregular blotches (circle). Excise this lesion.

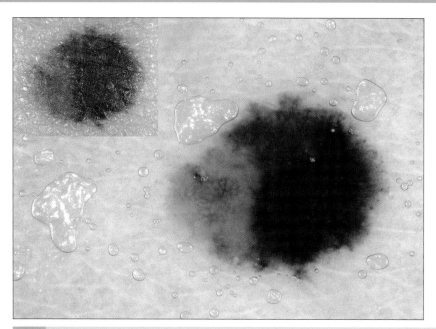

Figure 354 Melanoma

Imagination is needed to see the streaks and atypical pigment network that classify this as a reticular pattern. The dermoscopist should realize that this is a high-risk lesion because of the clearcut asymmetry of color and structure. As is the case here, an early in-situ melanoma may be hard to diagnose.

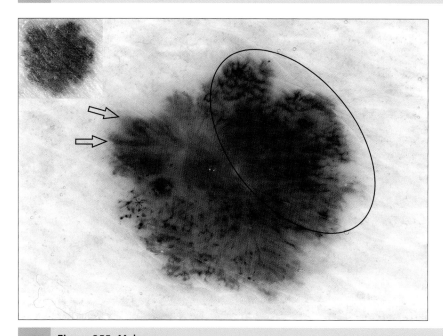

Figure 355 Melanoma

This bizarre dermoscopic picture shows areas with very atypical pigment network (circle), irregular streaks (arrows) and irregular dots and globules (asterisk). Never tell a patient that they definitely have a melanoma based on the dermoscopic picture, no matter how ominous it looks.

SPITZOID LESIONS

GENERAL PRINCIPLES

- Spitzoid means similar in appearance to a starburst pattern.
- Spitzoid differential diagnosis includes Clark (dysplastic) nevus, Spitz nevus and melanoma.
- Spitzoid morphology comprises a light-dark or blue central area and dots and globules or streaks at the periphery.
- Symmetrical spitzoid pattern = benign lesion.
- Asymmetrical spitzoid pattern – rule out melanoma.

- The stereotypical starburst pattern is seen more frequently than the globular pattern, which is more common than the non-specific spitzoid pattern.

CAUTION

Deaths have occurred secondary to metastatic 'Spitz' nevi that were in reality melanomas. Excise the vast majority of spitzoid lesions. It is better to be safe than sorry.

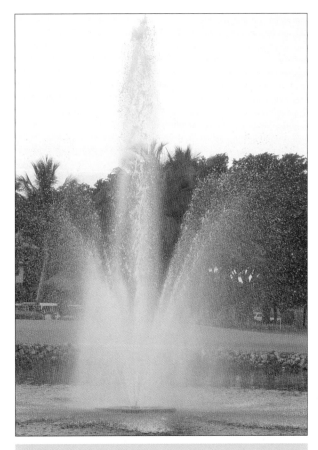

Starburst on a hot summer's day!

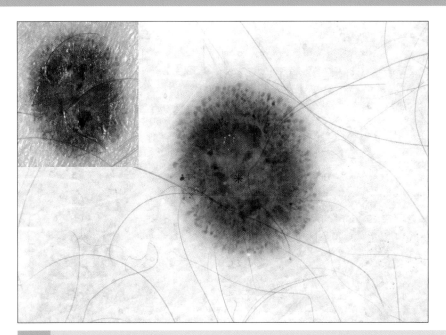

Figure 356 Spitz nevus

This is a classic symmetrical spitzoid pattern. In the center of the lesion there is a subtle blue-white structure (asterisk). The rim of dots and globules at all points along the periphery of the lesion allow this dermoscopic diagnosis. On looking carefully, there are also some streaks at the periphery.

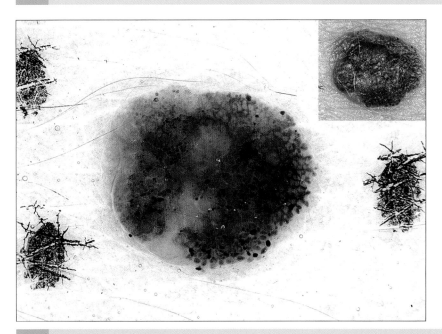

Figure 357 Melanoma

Compared to the lesion shown in Figure 356, this lesion demonstrates significant asymmetry of color and structure with several melanoma-specific criteria. Why then is this spitzoid? There is a central blue-white structure (asterisk) with irregular dots and globules and streaks at the periphery. They are trying to form a starburst pattern, but the criteria are not evenly distributed at the periphery of the lesion.

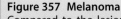

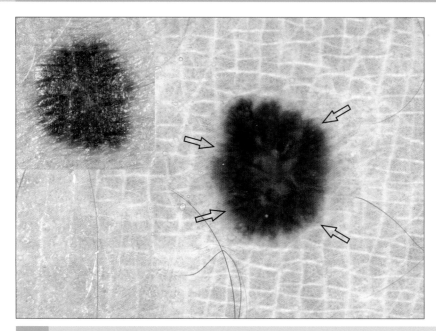

Figure 358 Spitz nevus
It is important to recognize symmetry and asymmetry in spitzoid lesions. This lesion is very symmetrical, with subtle radially oriented streaks (arrows) at all points along the periphery of the lesion. Remember the criteria are not always easy to see, so practice dermoscopy as much as possible to be able to see subtle patterns. The central blue-white structure is spitzoid.

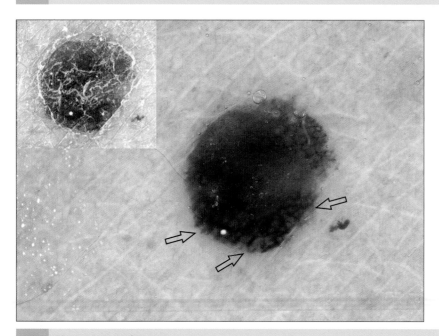

Figure 359 Melanoma
It is necessary to stretch one's imagination to call this a spitzoid nevus. It does fit the pattern because there is a central blue-white structure (asterisk) and there are asymmetrically located streaks (arrows) at the periphery. The pigment network is very atypical. It does not matter whether this is called spitzoid or not – it could be a melanoma and should be excised.

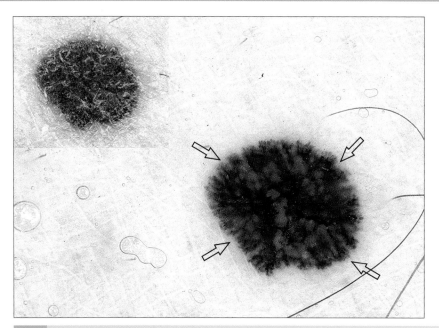

Figure 360 Spitz nevus

Here is another classic symmetrical starburst pattern. If this pattern is etched on the mind it will be recognized immediately. This Spitz nevus has a darker central blotch partially covering a blue-white structure, and symmetrically located streaks (arrows) at all points along the periphery of the lesion.

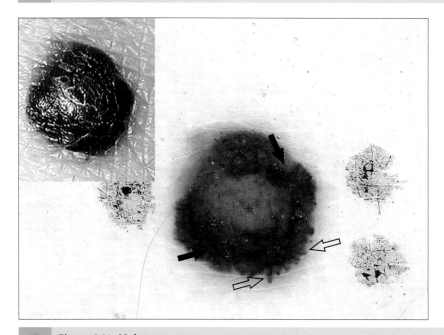

Figure 361 Melanoma

This is a spitzoid melanoma with a centrally located blue-white structure (asterisk), a horseshoe-shaped dark blotch (solid arrows) and asymmetrically located streaks (open arrows) at the periphery. Pink color – beware.

TAPE STRIPPING

GENERAL PRINCIPLES

- Tape stripping of flat lesions is a clinical tool to help uncover hidden dermoscopic criteria.
- The black lamella represents superficial pigmented parakeratotic cells that can be stripped away.
- Tape stripping can dramatically change a lesion's appearance.
- Tape stripping may not change the lesion at all.
- It takes only a minute to tape strip a flat black lesion. It is well worth the effort. At times the black color will be on the tape. Your patient will be impressed.

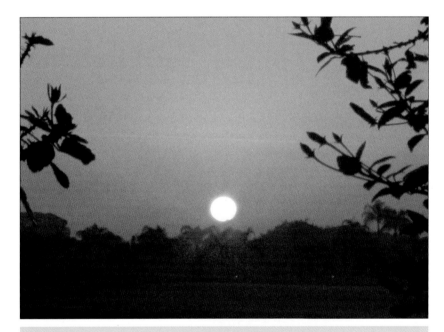

As night turns into day, everything will become easier to see.

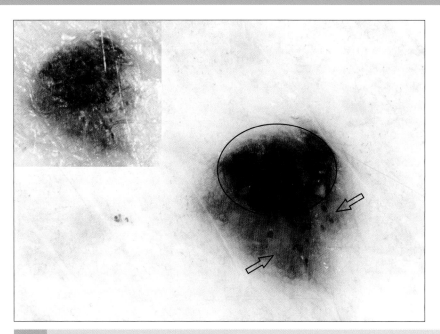

Figure 362 Clark (dysplastic) nevus
The image shows an asymmetrical lesion due to the presence of an irregular black blotch (circle) and irregular dots and globules (arrows).

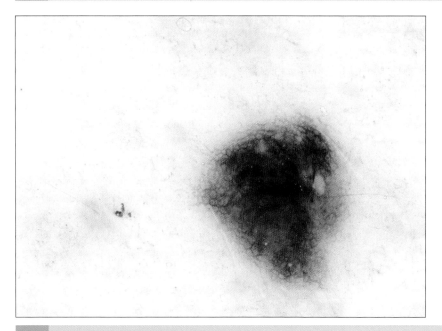

Figure 363 Clark (dysplastic) nevus
After tape stripping the black pigmentation seen in Figure 362 is completely removed and a regular pigment network is seen, allowing diagnosis of this Clark (dysplastic) nevus with confidence.

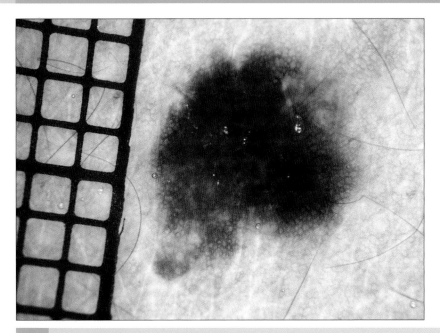

Figure 364 Clark (dysplastic) nevus

This is a worrisome-looking melanocytic lesion characterized by an asymmetrical distribution of colors and structures, an atypical pigment network, irregular black color and a blue-white structure (see Figure 365).

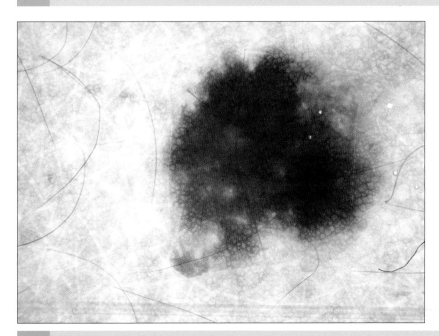

Figure 365 Clark (dysplastic) nevus

After tape stripping most of the black color partially covering the pigment network seen in Figure 364 is removed. However, the lesion remains asymmetrical because of an atypical pigment network. For this reason biopsy is needed.

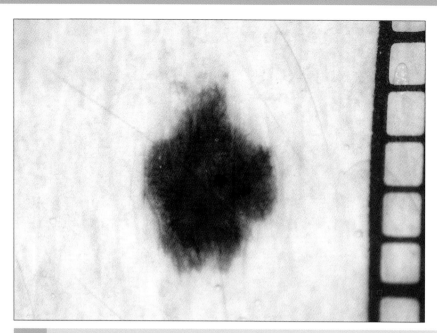

Figure 366 Clark (dysplastic) nevus
This lesion is the same as that in Figure 367 before tape stripping.

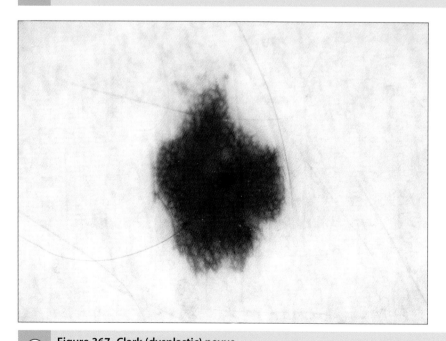

Figure 367 Clark (dysplastic) nevus
Once again, tape stripping has not dramatically changed this lesion, but it is looking less worrisome, with a typical pigment network being more evident. There is no increase in high-risk criteria such as streaks.

DIFFERENTIAL DIAGNOSTIC VALUE OF BLOOD VESSELS

GENERAL PRINCIPLES

- Blood vessels can be seen in melanocytic, non-melanocytic, benign and malignant lesions.
- Vessels can be seen with other criteria or vessels may be the only criterion found in a lesion.
- Some vessels are associated with high-risk pathology and others with low-risk pathology.
- Pink lesions with vessels may be melanocytic, non-melanocytic, benign or malignant. The shape of the vessels may provide a clue to the correct diagnosis.

MELANOCYTIC LESIONS

- Dermal nevi – comma-shaped vessels.
- Clark (dysplastic) nevi – comma-shaped and dotted vessels.
- Melanoma – dots and irregular linear vessels or milky-red areas.

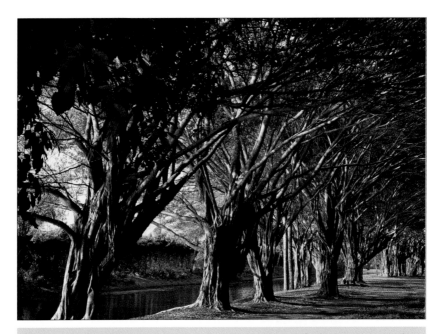

Such natural beauty should never be cut away, unless you find it in a patient's skin!

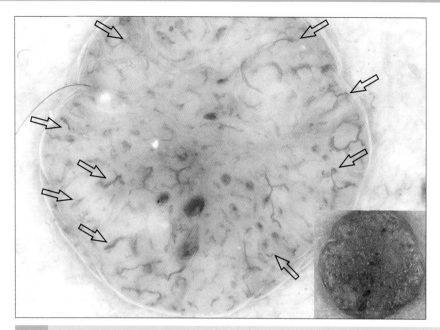

Figure 368 Dermal nevus

The correct diagnosis for this dermal nevus without pigmentation is suggested by the shape of the vessels. They are comma shaped (arrows). A few comedo-like openings, milia-like cysts and a hair follicle are also present. Do not confuse these vessels with the larger branching vessels seen in a basal cell carcinoma.

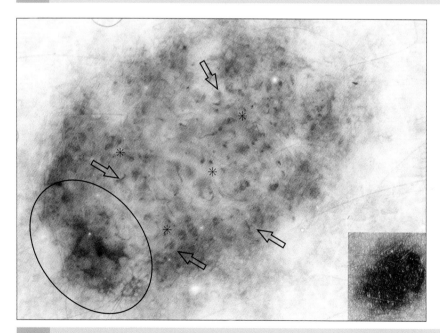

Figure 369 Clark (dysplastic) nevus

This lesion shows very subtle remnants of a pigment network and a few dots and globules (circle); therefore it is a melanocytic lesion. There is a combination of comma-shaped (arrows) and dotted (asterisks) vessels.

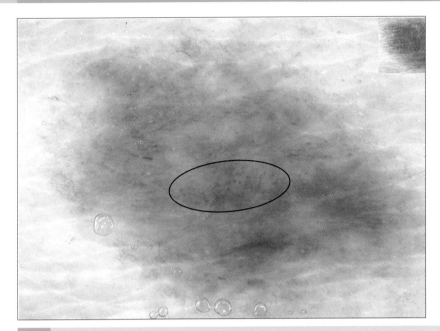

Figure 370 Spitz nevus
This lesion has a classic non-specific global pattern, so it could be high risk. Pink color – beware. It is a hypopigmented Spitz nevus with dotted and linear vessels (circle). The entire pinkish-white zone can also be called a milky-red area and is a high-risk vascular pattern. It is not always possible to differentiate dotted and linear vessels from milky-red areas, nor does it matter. A biopsy is indicated to rule out melanoma.

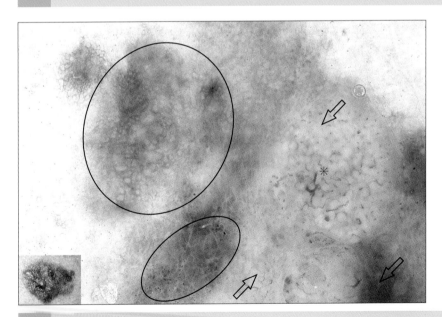

Figure 371 Melanoma
This lesion shows a multicomponent global pattern, which is commonly seen in melanomas. This is a hypopigmented melanoma with an atypical pigment network (upper circle), irregular subtle dots and globules (lower circle) and blue-white structures (arrows). The dotted and linear vessels (asterisk) are additional features of melanoma.

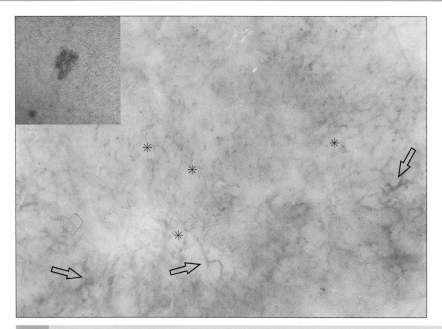

Figure 372 Melanoma

This is a dramatic 'featureless' amelanotic melanoma. Once seen it will never be forgotten. The lesion is flat and pinkish with dotted (asterisks) and irregular linear (arrows) vessels. Only a high index of suspicion will assure that this potentially deadly melanoma will not be missed.

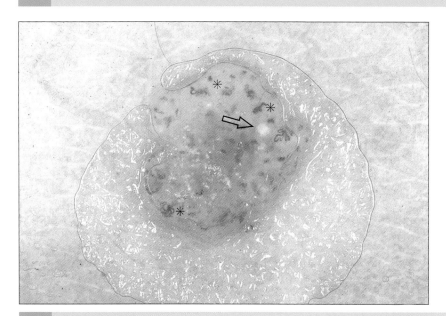

Figure 373 Melanoma

A milia-like cyst (arrow) does not make this a seborrheic keratosis. Dotted and irregular linear vessels (asterisks) would not be seen with a seborrheic keratosis. Even the most experienced dermoscopist might overlook this seemingly benign lesion. (Figure courtesy of MA Pizzichetta, Aviano, Italy.)

NON-MELANOCYTIC LESIONS

- Basal cell carcinoma – thick branching (arborizing) vessels.
- Seborrheic keratosis – hairpin shapes.
- Bowen's disease – small foci of dotted vessels that look like glomeruli in the kidney,

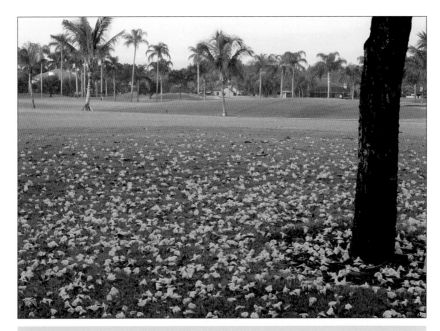

There are streaks, stereotypical milia-like cysts and pigmented follicular openings. Are you confused at this point? If so, go directly to Jail and do not pass Go!

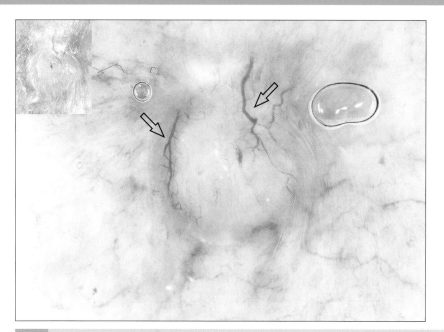

Figure 374 Basal cell carcinoma

This is a commonly seen basal cell carcinoma without pigment. The blood vessels, which are thick and branching (arrows), point to the correct diagnosis. The vessels are superficial and are therefore in focus. If the vessels are deeper in the lesion they would be blurred and out of focus. If so, think amelanotic melanoma.

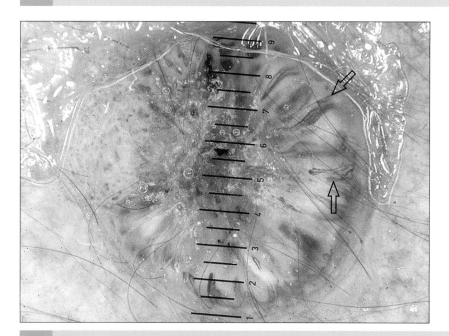

Figure 375 Keratoacanthoma

If there could be one, then this is a classic keratoacanthoma with hairpin-shaped vessels (arrows) and a white background. The white color is not always scarring seen with regression, but in this case represents hyperkeratosis seen in keratinizing tumors. White color can be seen in melanocytic, non-melanocytic, benign and malignant lesions. The central crust plus the history and clinical appearance all help in determining the management of this lesion.

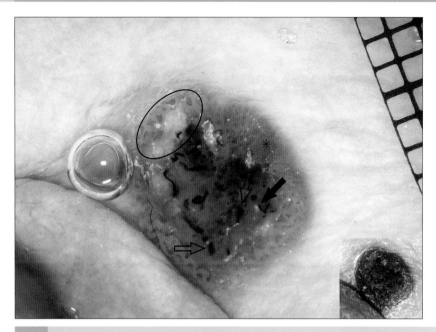

Figure 376 Seborrheic keratosis
This is an irritated seborrheic keratosis. The gray color (asterisk) represents pigmentary incontinence secondary to inflammation. Classic melanophages are not seen. Hairpin-shaped vessels (circle), a few milia-like cysts (closed arrow) and comedo-like openings (open arrows) can also be identified. This is a difficult lesion. If in doubt, cut it out!

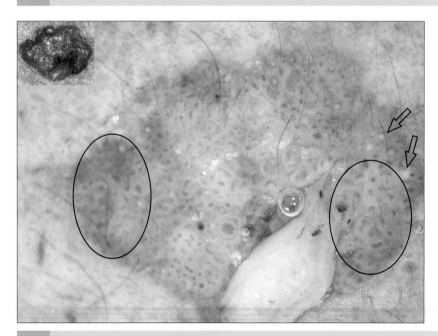

Figure 377 Seborrheic keratosis
This unusual non-pigmented seborrheic keratosis has hairpin-shaped vessels (circles) and a few milia-like cysts (arrows).

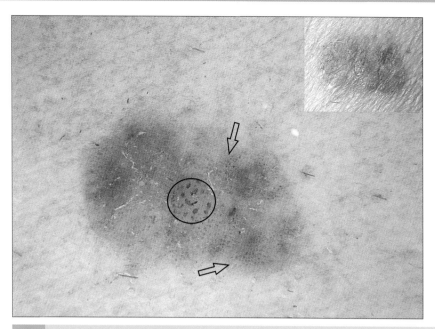

Figure 378 Bowen's disease

Pigmented Bowen's disease is a difficult clinical and dermoscopic diagnosis to make. It is usually a surprise to obtain this pathology report when in most cases a potentially high-risk melanocytic lesion has been suspected. Here there are well-circumscribed round areas of red vessels looking like a renal glomerulus (circle) and tiny brown dots packed together tightly (arrows).

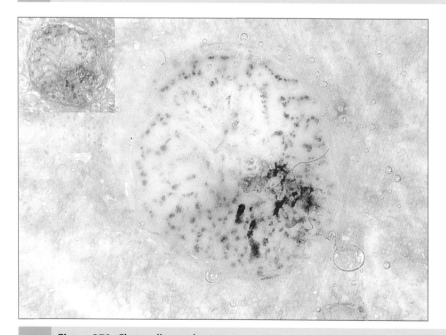

Figure 379 Clear cell acanthoma

Pink lesions with this pattern of dotted vessels as the only criteria are totally non-specific. The differential diagnosis includes melanocytic, non-melanocytic, benign and malignant lesions. If there is only one lesion, excise it. The presence of several lesions points to low-risk pathology. Biopsy one to make a dermoscopic–pathologic correlation.

DIAGNOSTIC PEARLS

- Don't jump to conclusions.
- You can't see what you do not know. The more you study or practice, the better you will be.
- Dermoscopy is not a 100% diagnostic technique. Don't expect it to be.
- Evaluate all criteria before making a dermoscopic diagnosis.
- Gut feelings about a lesion are important and should not be ignored.
- Don't be discouraged if you make a mistake. We all do and it will be a learning experience that will improve your dermoscopic skills.
- Don't forget the importance of the patient's personal and family history, as well as the clinical appearance and history of the lesion you are examining.
- Look for subtle high-risk criteria before diagnosing a lesion as being low risk.
- Always have a dermoscopic differential diagnosis.
- When possible make a dermoscopic clinicopathologic correlation.
- Don't hesitate to ask a more experienced colleague for his or her dermoscopic opinion.
- Use the most atypical dermoscopic area if you plan an incisional biopsy.
- Do not hesitate to seek a second opinion if you do not have a good dermoscopic clinicopathologic correlation with high-risk lesions.
- Give a hirsute patient a haircut to get a better look at a suspicious lesion.
- If the patient has dry skin and the dryness is on the lesion you are examining, get rid of the dryness and then check the lesion.
- A soft, compressible lesion favors low-risk pathology. Don't hesitate to palpate a lesion that you are concerned about.
- Recent sun exposure can make things look bad. Recheck the patient in a few weeks' time.
- If in doubt cut it out!

Further Reading

Akasu R, Sugiyama H, Araki M, Ohtake N, Furue M, Tamaki K. Dermatoscopic and videomicroscopic features of melanocytic plantar nevi. Am J Dermatopathol 1996;18:10–8.

Argenyi ZB. Dermoscopy (epiluminescence microscopy) of pigmented skin lesions. Current status and evolving trends. Dermatol Clin 1997;15:79–95.

Argenziano G, Fabbrocini G, Carli P, De Giorgi V, Sammarco E, Delfino M. Epiluminescence microscopy for the diagnosis of doubtful melanocytic skin lesions. Comparison of the ABCD rule of dermatoscopy and a new 7-point checklist based on pattern analysis. Arch Dermatol 1998;134:1563–70.

Argenziano G, Scalvenzi M, Staibano S, Brunetti B, Piccolo D, Delfino M, et al. Dermatoscopic pitfalls in differentiating pigmented Spitz naevi from cutaneous melanomas. Br J Dermatol 1999;141:788–93.

Argenziano G, Soyer HP, Chimenti S, Ruocco V. Impact of dermoscopy on the clinical management of pigmented skin lesions. Clin Dermatol 2002;20:200–2.

Argenziano G, Soyer HP, Chimenti S, Talamini R, Corona R, Sera F, et al. Dermoscopy of pigmented skin lesions: Results of a consensus meeting via the Internet. J Am Acad Dermatol. 2003;48:679–93.

Argenziano G, Soyer HP, DeGiorgi V, et al. Interactive atlas of dermoscopy (Book and CD-ROM). Milan: EDRA-Medical Publishing & New Media, 2000.

Argenziano G, Soyer HP. Dermoscopy of pigmented skin lesions–a valuable tool for early diagnosis of melanoma. Lancet Oncol 2001;2:443–9.

Bafounta ML, Beauchet A, Aegerter P, Saiag P. Is dermoscopy (epiluminescence microscopy) useful for the diagnosis of melanoma? Results of a meta-analysis using techniques adapted to the evaluation of diagnostic tests. Arch Dermatol 2001;137:1343–50.

Bauer J, Metzler G, Rassner G, et al. Dermatoscopy turns histopathologists attention to the suspicious area in melanocytic lesions. Arch Dermatol 2001; 137:1338–1340

Binder M, Puespoeck-Schwarz M, Steiner A, Kittler H, Muellner M, Wolff K, et al. Epiluminescence microscopy of small pigmented skin lesions: short-term formal training improves the diagnostic performance of dermatologists. J Am Acad Dermatol 1997;36:197–202.

Binder M, Schwarz M, Winkler A, Steiner A, Kaider A, Wolff K, et al. Epiluminescence microscopy. A useful tool for the diagnosis of pigmented skin lesions for formally trained dermatologists. Arch Dermatol 1995;131:286–91.

Braun RP, Rabinovitz H, Kopf AW, et al. Dermoscopic diagnosis of seborrheic keratosis. Clin Dermatol 2002; 20:270–272.

Braun RP, Rabinovitz HS, Kopf AW, et al. Pattern Analysis: A two-step procedure for the dermoscopic diagnosis of melanoma. Clinics in Dermatology 2002; 20:236–239

Carli P, De Giorgi V, Giannotti B. Dermoscopy and early diagnosis of melanoma: the light and the dark. Arch Dermatol 2001;137:1641–4.

Carli P, De Giorgi V, Naldi L, Dosi G. Reliability and inter-observer agreement of dermoscopic diagnosis of melanoma and melanocytic naevi. Dermoscopy Panel. Eur J Cancer Prev 1998;7:397–402.

Carli P, Massi D, DeGiorgi V, Giannotti B. Clinically and dermoscopically featureless melanoma: When prevention fails. J Am Acad Dermatol 2002; 46:957–9

Ferrara G, Argenziano G, Soyer HP, Corona R, Sera F, Brunetti B, et al. Dermoscopic and histopathologic diagnosis of equivocal melanocytic skin lesions: an interdisciplinary study on 107 cases. Cancer 2002;95:1094–100.

Friedman RJ, Rigel DS, Silverman MK, et al. Malignant melanoma in the 1990's: The continued importance of early detection and the role of physician examination and self-examination of the skin. CA Cancer J Clin 1991; 41:201–226

Grin CM, Friedman KP, Grant-Kels JM. Dermoscopy: a review. Dermatol Clin 2002;20:641–6.

Grob JJ, Bonerandi JJ. The 'ugly duckling' sign: identification of the common characteristics of nevi in an individual as a basis for melanoma screening. Arch Dermatol 1998; 134:103–4

Hofmann-Wellenhof R, Blum A, Wolf IH, Piccolo D, Kerl H, Garbe C, et al. Dermoscopic classification of atypical melanocytic nevi (Clark nevi). Arch Dermatol 2001;137:1575–80.

Johr R, Izakovic J. Should you be using epiluminescence microscopy? Skin Aging, March 2000:28–38

Johr RH, Izakovic J. Dermatoscopy/ELM for the evaluation of nail-apparatus pigmentation. Dermatol Surg 2001;27:315–22.

Johr RH, Schachner LA, Izakovic J. Lessons on dermoscopy #8. A high-risk melanocytic lesion. Dermatol Surg 2000;26:893–5.

Johr RH, Stolz W. Lentigo maligna and lentigo maligna melanoma. J Am Acad Dermatol 1997;37:512

Johr RH, Stolz W. Lesions in Dermoscopy 'milky-red' areas. Dermatol Surg 2002; 28:299–300

Johr RH. Dermoscopy: alternative melanocytic algorithms-the ABCD rule of dermatoscopy, Menzies scoring method, and 7-point checklist. Clin Dermatol 2002;20:240–7.

Johr RH. Pink lesions. Clin Dermatol 2002; 20:189–296.

Kenet RO, Kang S, Kenet BJ, Fitzpatrick TB, Sober AJ, Barnhill RL. Clinical diagnosis of pigmented lesions using digital epiluminescence microscopy. Grading protocol and atlas. Arch Dermatol 1993;129:157–74.

Kenet RO, Kenet BJ. Risk stratification. A practical approach to using epiluminescence microscopy/dermoscopy in melanoma screening. Dermatol Clin 2001;19:327–35.

Kittler H, Binder M. Follow-up of Melanocytic Skin Lesions With Digital Dermoscopy: Risks and Benefits. Arch Dermatol 2002;138:1379.

Kittler H, Pehamberger H, Wolff K, Binder M. Diagnostic accuracy of dermoscopy. Lancet Oncol 2002;3:159–65.

Kittler H, Pehamberger H, Wolff K, Binder M. Follow-up of melanocytic skin lesions with digital epiluminescence microscopy: patterns of modifications observed in early melanoma, atypical nevi, and common nevi. J Am Acad Dermatol 2000;43:467–76.

Kittler H, Seltenheim M, Dawid M, Pehamberger H, Wolff K, Binder M. Frequency and characteristics of enlarging common melanocytic nevi. Arch Dermatol 2000;136:316–20.

Kreusch JF. Vascular patterns in skin tumors. Clin Dermatol 2002; 20:248–254.

Lorentzen HF, Weismann K Secher L, et al. The dermatoscopic ABCD rule does not improve diagnostic accuracy of malignant melanoma. Acta Derm Venereol 2000; 80:223

Lorentzen HF, Weismann K, Larsen FG. Structural asymmetry as a dermatoscopic indicator of malignant melanoma: a latent class analysis of sensitivity and classification errors. Melanoma Res 2001; 11:495–501

Mayer J. Systematic review of the diagnostic accuracy of dermatoscopy in detecting malignant melanoma. Med J Aust 1997;167:206–10.

Menzies SW, Crotty KA, Ingvar C, McCarthy WM. An atlas of surface microscopy of pigmented skin lesions: Dermoscopy. McGraw-Hill 2003.

Menzies SW, Gutenev A, Avramidis M, Batrac A, McCarthy WH. Short-term digital surface microscopic monitoring of atypical or changing melanocytic lesions. Arch Dermatol 2001;137:1583–9.

Menzies SW, Ingvar C, Crotty KA, McCarthy WH. Frequency and morphologic characteristics of invasive melanomas lacking specific surface microscopic features. Arch Dermatol 1996;132:1178–82.

Menzies SW, Ingvar C, McCarthy WH. A sensitivity and specificity analysis of the surface microscopy features of invasive melanoma. Melanoma Res 1996; 6:55–62

Menzies SW, Westerhoff K, Rabinovitz H, Kopf AW, McCarthy WH, Katz B. Surface microscopy of pigmented basal cell carcinoma. Arch Dermatol 2000;136(8):1012–6.

Menzies SW. A method for the diagnosis of primary cutaneous melanoma using surface microscopy. Dermatol Clin 2001; 19:299–305.

Pagnanelli G, Soyer HP, Argenziano G, Talamini R, Barbati R, Bianchi L, et al. Diagnosis of pigmented skin lesions by dermoscopy: web-based training improves diagnostic performance of non-experts. Br J Dermatol 2003;148:698–702.

Pehamberger H, Binder M, Steiner A, Wolff K. In vivo epiluminescence microscopy: improvement of early diagnosis of melanoma. J Invest Dermatol 1993; 100(Suppl): 356–625

Pehamberger H, Steiner A, Wolff K. In vivo epiluminescence microscopy of pigmented skin lesions. I. Pattern analysis of pigmented skin lesions. J Am Acad Dermatol 1987;17:571–83.

Peris K, Ferrari A, Argenziano G, Soyer HP, et al. Dermoscopic classification of Spitz/Reed nevi. Clin Dermatol 2002; 20:259–262

Pizzichetta MA, Talamini R, Piccolo D, et al. The ABCD rule of dermatoscopy does not apply to small melanocytic skin lesions. Arch Dermatol 2001; 137:1376–8

Rabinovitz H, Kopfa AW, Katz B: Dermoscopy: A practical guide. CD rom version. mm A Worldwide Group Inc. 1999.

Ronger S, Touzet S, Ligeron C, Balme B, Viallard AM, Barrut D, et al. Dermoscopic examination of nail pigmentation. Arch Dermatol 2002;138:1327–33.

Saida T, Oguchi S, Ishihara Y. In vivo observation of magnified features of pigmented lesions on volar skin using video macroscope. Usefulness of epiluminescence techniques in clinical diagnosis. Arch Dermatol 1995;131:298–304.

Saida T, Oguchi S, Miyazaki A. Dermoscopy for acral pigmented skin lesions. Clin Dermatol 2002;20:279–85.

Salopek TG, Kopf AW, Stetanoto CM, et al. Differentiation of atypical moles (dysplastic nevi) from early melanoma by dermoscopy. Dermatol Clin 2001; 19:337–45

Schiffner R, Schiffner-Rohe J, Vogt T, Landthaler M, Wlotzke U, Cognetta AB, et al. Improvement of early recognition of lentigo maligna using dermatoscopy. J Am Acad Dermatol 2000;42:25–32.

Seidenari S, Pellacani G. Surface Microscopy features of congenital nevi. Clin Dermatol 2002; 20:263–267.

Soyer HP, Argenziano G, Chimenti S, et al. Dermoscopy of pigmented skin lesions: an atlas based on the Consensus Net Meeting on Dermoscopy 2000. Milan: EDRA Medical Publishing and New Media. 2001

Soyer HP, Argenziano G, Chimenti S, Ruocco V. Dermoscopy of pigmented skin lesions. Eur J Dermatol 2001;11:270–7.

Soyer HP, Argenziano G, Ruocco V, Chimenti S. Dermoscopy of pigmented skin lesions (Part II). Eur J Dermatol 2001;11:483–98.

Soyer HP, Argenziano G, Talamini R, Chimenti S. Is dermoscopy useful for the diagnosis of melanoma? Arch Dermatol 2001;137:1361–3.

Soyer HP, Kenet RO, Wolf IH, Kenet BJ, Cerroni L. Clinicopathological correlation of pigmented skin lesions using dermoscopy. Eur J Dermatol 2000;10:22–8.

Soyer HP, Smolle J, Hodl S, Pachernegg H, Kerl H. Surface microscopy. A new approach to the diagnosis of cutaneous pigmented tumors. Am J Dermatopathol 1989;11:1–10.

Soyer HP, Smolle J, Leitinger G, Rieger E, Kerl H. Diagnostic reliability of dermoscopic criteria for detecting malignant melanoma. Dermatology 1995;190:25–30.

Steiner A, Binder M, Schemper M, et al. Statistical evaluation of epiluminescence microscopic criteria for melanocytic pigmented skin lesions. J Am Acad Dermatol 1993;29:581

Steiner A, Pehamberger H, Binder M, Wolff K. Pigmented Spitz nevi: improvement of the diagnostic accuracy by epiluminescence microscopy. J Am Acad Dermatol 1992; 27:697–701

Steiner A, Pehamberger H, Wolff K. In vivo epiluminescence microscopy of pigmented skin lesions. II. Diagnosis of small pigmented skin lesions and early detection of malignant melanoma. J Am Acad Dermatol 1987;17:584–91.

Stolz W, Braun-Falco O, Bilek P, et al. Color atlas of dermatoscopy. 2nd ed. Oxford, England: Blackwell Scientific Publications, 2002

Stolz W, Schiffner R, Burgdorf WH. Dermatoscopy for facial pigmented skin lesions. Clin Dermatol 2002;20:276–8.

Tosti A, Argenziano G. Dermoscopy allows better management of nail pigmentation. Arch Dermatol 2002;138:1369–70.

Tripp JM, Kopf AW, Marghoob AA et al. Management of dysplastic nevi: A survey of fellows of the American Academy of Dermatology. J Am Acad Dermatol 2002; 46:674–82

Westerhoff K, McCarthy WH, Menzies SW. Increase in the sensitivity for melanoma diagnosis by primary care physicians using skin surface microscopy. Br J Dermatol 2000;143:1016–20.

Wolf I. Dermoscopic diagnosis of vascular lesions. Clin Dermatol 2002; 20:273–275.

Wolff K. Why is epiluminescence microscopy important? Recent Results Cancer Res 2002;160:125–32.

www.dermoscopy.org Consensus Net Meeting on Dermoscopy (CNMD) 2000. Unifying concepts of Dermoscopy.

Yadav S, Vossaert KA, Kopf AW, Silverman M, Grin-Jorgensen C. Histopathologic correlates of structures seen on dermoscopy (epiluminescence microscopy). Am J Dermatopathol 1993;15:297–305.

Index